How to Succeed at Medical School

An essential guide to learning

Dedication

To Geert and Jerry, for their support and patience,
without which this book would never have been written.

How to Succeed at Medical School

An essential guide to learning

Dason Evans
Head of Clinical Skills
Centre for Medical and Healthcare Education
St George's, University of London
London, UK

Jo Brown
Senior Lecturer in Clinical Communication
Centre for Medical and Healthcare Education
St George's, University of London
London, UK

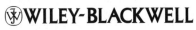

A John Wiley & Sons, Ltd., Publication

This edition first published 2009, © 2009 by Dason Evans and Jo Brown

BMJ Books is an imprint of BMJ Publishing Group Limited, used under licence by Blackwell Publishing which was acquired by John Wiley & Sons in February 2007. Blackwell's publishing programme has been merged with Wiley's global Scientific, Technical and Medical business to form Wiley-Blackwell.

Registered office: John Wiley & Sons Ltd, The Atrium, Southern Gate, Chichester, West Sussex, PO19 8SQ, UK

Editorial offices: 9600 Garsington Road, Oxford, OX4 2DQ, UK
The Atrium, Southern Gate, Chichester, West Sussex, PO19 8SQ, UK
111 River Street, Hoboken, NJ 07030-5774, USA

For details of our global editorial offices, for customer services and for information about how to apply for permission to reuse the copyright material in this book please see our website at www.wiley.com/wiley-blackwell

Library of Congress Cataloging-in-Publication Data
Evans, Dason.
How to succeed at medical school : an essential guide to learning / Dason Evans, Jo Brown.
p. ; cm.
Includes index.
ISBN: 978-1-4051-5139-9
1. Medical education.   2. Medical students.   3. Medical colleges.   4. Learning.
I. Brown, Jo, 1957–   II. Title.
[DNLM: 1. Education, Medical–methods.   2. Learning. W 18 E916h 2009]
R737.E93 2009
610.71′1–dc22

2008033371

ISBN: 978-1-4051-5139-9

A catalogue record for this book is available from the British Library.

Set in 9.5/12 Minion by Graphicraft Limited, Hong Kong
Printed and bound in Great Britain by TJ International Ltd, Padstow, Cornwall

4   2011

Contents

About the Authors

Dason Evans and Jo Brown have worked together on and off since 2000, initially at Bart's and the London School of Medicine and Dentistry where they were awarded the Drapers Prize "in recognition of the exemplary practice and innovation for enhancing the quality of learning and teaching", and more recently at St George's, University of London, where they have been appointed joint Chief Examiners for OSCEs. They have an international reputation for their work supporting students in academic difficulty and this expertise brings insights to this book which will benefit all students. They are recognised for their student-centred approach to learning and their passionate advocacy for the need to empower students to make the best use of the learning opportunities open to them.

Dr Dason Evans is a Senior Lecturer in medical education and head of clinical skills at St George's, University of London. He is following a career in medical education and works clinically in sexual health. He has been working formally in medical education since 1999 and teaching and supporting students since 1995. Dr Evans has strong interests in clinical skills learning, teaching and assessment, and learning within the clinical environment. Through his fellowship of the Higher Education Academy (HEA), and active contribution to the Association for the Study of Medical Education (ASME) and the Association for Medical Education in Europe (AMEE) and external examining duties he has a clear understanding of the current culture in health professional education. His research interests include clinical skills, preparation for practice, students in academic difficulty and education around sexual health.

Jo Brown is a Senior Lecturer in Clinical Communication at St George's, University of London. She started her career in nursing and management and has been teaching medical students, management students and nursing students since 1992. She has taught clinical communication since 1998 and her enthusiasm for the subject is infectious. She is a curriculum designer, a responsible examiner and external examiner for OSCEs. She is an experienced mentor for new teachers in higher education and runs courses for those teaching clinical communication using experiential learning techniques. She is a member of the UK Council of Communication Skills Teaching in Undergraduate Medical Education, the Medical Interview Teaching Association (MITA), ASME and is a fellow of the HEA. Her research interests currently centre around the transfer of learning from classroom to clinical environment and the challenges to learning in the clinical workplace.

Foreword

Throughout the working career of a doctor keeping up to date is a major factor in providing good care to patients. This book aims to help undergraduates learn some of the huge number of different skills required to distil new facts and new knowledge in order to keep ahead with their learning for the rest of their professional life. It is a most unusual book in that it is written to help students develop their own skills and awareness around learning. It does not contain factual knowledge but is about the skills required to cope with medical school. It covers aspects of learning such as cognitive skills, motivation, self-regulation of study skills, and the actual 'concept' of learning rather than the content for knowledge. It helps aid students to learn effectively and efficiently and even tells you how you will know when you know enough!

It does this in sections about knowledge, learning clinical and communication skills, learning how to work in a small group and, lastly, it even gives helpful advice on 'examination technique'! There are helpful suggestions about reflecting on the type of learner the student is and how to revise for examinations. Above all, it discusses the broader issues about 'living' and how to achieve a good life–work balance. It also helps with the aspirations of students and guides them to think about the future and the type of career they might like.

Although the authors say that they have written this book for students about to embark on a medical course and younger medical students, this book would also help those involved in 'teaching' healthcare professionals. It certainly would have saved me a lot of time learning how to get through a medical course.

The authors both have a vast experience in this area and much of their book has been gleaned from first-hand experience. I certainly enjoyed reading it and would recommend it to all students and teachers.

Parveen Kumar
Professor of Medicine and Education,
Barts and the London School of Medicine and Dentistry,
Queen Mary College,
University of London

Introduction

Who is this book for?

You may be reading this book because you are thinking of joining a medical course, or because you are in the first few years of training. In this case you will find this book particularly useful in helping you manage the transition to new ways of learning. This book will also be of interest to more senior students, and may be of interest and relevance to students of other health professions and academics involved in their learning.

What is this book for?

Learning how to learn effectively and efficiently

During your years at medical school you will buy plenty of books. Almost all these books will cover *what* you need to know. This book is different, it concentrates on *how to learn effectively and efficiently* whilst at medical school and beyond. There is good evidence that helping students develop their awareness of how to learn, and helping them develop a variety of learning techniques results in large improvements in performance.

Medical school is different

The learning environment at medical school is fundamentally different to secondary school or other university courses. You are expected to learn a huge amount of diverse information, ranging from Anatomy to Ethics, to become proficient in many new skills, ranging from taking blood to breaking bad news, and to be able to integrate skills with knowledge in order to work with a patient to make a diagnosis and management plan. You are expected to learn much of this without being specifically taught it. You are expected to be able to find out what you need to know, and to learn it to an appropriate level, often with little support.

How to Succeed at Medical School: an essential guide to learning. By Dason Evans and Jo Brown. Published 2009 by Blackwell Publishing, ISBN: 978-1-4051-5139-9.

How will this book help you?

This book works on two levels. On the first level it offers advice on how to learn most efficiently (study skills). This is divided up into four sections: *learning knowledge, learning clinical and communication skills, working in a group* and *exam technique*. On the second level it aims to get you thinking about how you learn, and when it might be best to use which study skills. This is embedded within these four sections, and covered in more depth in four other sections: "what kind of learner are you?", "life–work balance", "revision" and "thinking ahead." By reading and working through this book you will gain not only a wider range of study skills, but also an awareness of when to use them in your learning.

What is in it?

An overview of the sections

The book starts with a chapter called *What kind of learner are you?* which introduces a simple overview of learning style, and helps you to think about what your preferred learning style is, and how this might influence your learning. For example you may be a perfectionist, wanting to understand the deepest nuances of everything that you learn – if this is the case you may have trouble knowing at which point what you have learned is good enough, and when to move on to the next thing to learn. In contrast you might be a crammer, great at filling your head with facts for a few weeks before your exams, ready to forget shortly after – if this is the case, the volume of study may well overwhelm you, however good your short-term memory.

The chapter on *Learning knowledge* covers how to make the most of lectures, including taking lecture notes; what sort of books to use and how to learn from them, including note taking, reviewing your learning and testing yourself; how to sift out the rubbish from the internet and search effectively using IT; making the most of the library; how to find appropriate review articles from journals that give the most up-to-date view.

In the chapters on *Learning Clinical skills* and *Clinical Communication skills*, we offer guidance on how to be self-directed in learning these skills, how to make the most out of simulation and how to capitalise on the richness that learning with patients offers. We specifically cover the clinical learning environment, as many students find the clinical setting (hospital wards, general practice) a very different and unstructured environment to learn in, we discuss how to get the most from your clinical tutors and where some of the hidden learning opportunities are. With respect to clinical communication skills we present an evidence based approach and advice on learning both in simulation and in the clinical environment: learning both by doing, but also by watching others. Finally we discuss feedback, both how to give effective feedback, and also how to receive it, to act on it.

Much of the learning in medical schools in the UK is through *Working in a group*. Working and learning in a group is inescapable in medicine, and this section starts with a discussion on the pros and cons of group work, and how to get the best from it. It specifically discusses Problem Based Learning (PBL) and its variants, informal learning groups and how to make interprofessional learning work.

Students at medical school often struggle with developing an *Academic writing* style, referencing appropriately and concepts of plagiarism. We give an introduction to these areas in a dedicated chapter which we hope will start you off with safe foundations.

Portfolios and reflection are inescapable in undergraduate and postgraduate medical education, and the chapter on the subject gives a pragmatic overview on what portfolios are and how to make them work for you, and demystifies some of the concepts of reflection.

For the rest of your life, there will be too much to do at work, and too much to do at home. Balancing social and professional lives forms a recurring theme in research about stress in doctors. The chapter on *Life-work balance* provides some guidance into how to manage both a healthy social life and a healthy study life, and, most importantly, will help you get into good habits right at the start of your professional career. Both time management and stress management are covered here.

The chapter on *Revision* builds on and summarises the principles from the previous ones, discussing how to manage the learning environment, prioritising, planning and timetabling, and managing stress. This chapter above all others offers wholesome, sensible advice on how to manage the limited time running up to exams.

The chapters on *Exam technique* cover generic advice about how to approach exams, lists the different kinds of assessments that you might face at medical school and then offers specific advice on how to make the most from each of these. It includes how to do your best in multiple choice and extended matching question exams, how to survive the OSCE or clinical skills exam and discusses coping mechanisms that don't work, alongside those that do, and advice on how to manage exam stress.

Finally, the chapter on *Thinking ahead: Selected study components, Careers and Electives* offers some thoughts about longer term planning of learning – including which optional components of your course to choose, which electives to go on, and some discussion on how to check out what career in medicine might be right for you.

A word about professionalism

You might notice flicking through the chapter titles that something seems to be missing. There is no chapter on professionalism, and at first glance this might seem strange. Professionalism is the very foundation of medical practice and this is mirrored in this book. Professionalism is not separate, but integrated within each chapter. Whether it be learning effectively, encouraging life-long learning, concepts of referencing and plagiarism or a strong emphasis on learning in order to provide excellent care for patients, rather than to pass exams, you will find little in this book that will not count toward your developing professionalism.

How to use this book

This book has been written to provide a whole view, but each chapter has been designed to stand alone, with considerable cross referencing. Whether you prefer to start at the beginning and read start to finish or dip in and out, both approaches will work. We highly recommend that you read with some rough paper handy and *actively engage* with the few exercises that you will find in most chapters – it will be easy to skip them, but your understanding and learning will not be as deep if you do. Teaching on learning styles (what kind of learner are you) and on life work balance are often unappealing. We have worked hard to make these chapters relevant, interesting and practical, they are fundamental and we would strongly encourage you to give them a go.

Summary

This book will not teach you what you need to know to be a doctor. However, by using this book actively you *will* learn how to study more effectively and efficiently at medical school, how to balance this study with an enjoyable social life, and how to show your best abilities in the exams. In other words, this book will show you how to thrive at medical school and how to enjoy learning for the rest of your life.

Chapter 1 **What kind of learner are you?**

OVERVIEW

This chapter forms a foundation for the rest of this book. It will help you become aware of your learning preferences, and the factors that tend to affect your learning. This awareness itself will be useful to you, both with respect to planning your learning and with respect to highlighting which chapters of the book you are likely to find particularly important. We have tried to give a brief overview of the most important factors, and have tried to encourage you to make some judgements. You might want to revisit this chapter when you have finished the book to see if your impressions have changed.

Introduction

This chapter might be quite tough to work through. It asks you to take time away from reading to think about the things that affect your learning. The temptation will be just to read on; however, you will benefit considerably from having a few sheets of paper handy and trying to answer each question. Concentrate on each brief exercise and answer it as best you can, it will make the information sink in much better. At the end of the chapter we have put a summary diagram, which we hope will highlight where you have assessed your strengths and weaknesses.

We will cover the following aspects of learning:

- cognitive aspects (how deep is your learning?)
- motivation (what drives you to learn?)
- self-regulation of study skills (are you aware of how you learn?)
- how do you know when you know enough?
- conception of learning (what you think learning is for)

How to Succeed at Medical School: an essential guide to learning. By Dason Evans and Jo Brown. Published 2009 by Blackwell Publishing, ISBN: 978-1-4051-5139-9.

- learning in groups (love it or hate it)
- mood and learning (a help or a hindrance)
- VARK (your preferences in using your senses in learning)

You may want to have a brief break after each section, as there is quite a bit to think about.

Aspects of learning

You may have already completed learning style inventories or psychometric tests to try and define what sort of learner you are. There are all sorts of different learning styles that each tend to look at slightly different aspects of learning. The authors of the learning styles inventories claim that greatness can be reached by understanding how you think and learn, using their learning style inventory of course. Our aim is more modest – we hope that by thinking about how you learn, you will become aware of what aspects of learning you will find easier, and where the challenges might lie ahead for you.

> *Filling in a learning style questionnaire was fantastic, it helped me realise the kind of learner I am and build on my natural style.*
>
> Jo, first-year graduate entry student

Cognitive aspects
This refers to the way that you go about building new information into memories – how much do you skim over the surface or how much do you struggle to really understand, how well can you remember something that you have learned? For how long?

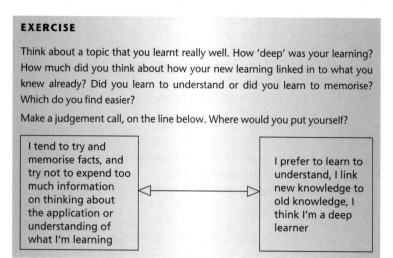

EXERCISE

Think about a topic that you learnt really well. How 'deep' was your learning? How much did you think about how your new learning linked in to what you knew already? Did you learn to understand or did you learn to memorise? Which do you find easier?

Make a judgement call, on the line below. Where would you put yourself?

I tend to try and memorise facts, and try not to expend too much information on thinking about the application or understanding of what I'm learning

I prefer to learn to understand, I link new knowledge to old knowledge, I think I'm a deep learner

If you have a preference for memorisation (the left-hand end of the line), then you will do very well with some things – drug names, anatomy, tests that ask you to regurgitate facts – but you are likely to struggle more on those tasks that require a deep understanding or application of the facts; unfortunately, a good amount of research indicates that students scoring towards the right tend to do better at medical school. You might think about some strategies to encourage you to shift more to the right, and in Chapter 2 (learning knowledge) we will go through some of these. If you tend to memorise as many facts as possible shortly before exams, forgetting them shortly after, and have an easy time the rest of the year, then you will run into trouble with the volume of work in medicine, and will need to start working regularly; this might be a challenge for you.

We give more tips on encouraging deep learning in Chapter 2, and advice on timetabling and regular study in Chapter 8.

Motivation

What makes you learn? Do you learn for interest, or perhaps to pass exams, or even to please others? Some medical students learn best because they are fascinated by the science of medicine, others learn best when they can see the practical application of their learning, and a few learn best when someone is standing over them pressurising them.

EXERCISE

Spend a minute thinking about what motivates your learning. You might want to spend some time talking with your friends about this, be honest with yourself. As you come to a decision, think about how you might make use of this insight.

I am most motivated to learn by:

- If you find the science fascinating, spend a couple of hours each week in the library looking at the journals – *Nature*, the *Lancet*. When learning about diabetes, you will want to read about insulin receptors, about the pathology, about the underlying mechanisms by which diabetes causes increased cardiovascular risk, in addition to the core areas that you *need* to learn. The commonest pitfall if you are this kind of learner is that you might have some trouble with knowing when to stop reading, and when enough is enough – you cannot have a PhD level of knowledge on everything in medicine; we discuss tactics to manage this in Chapter 2.

- If it is patients and the practical application of knowledge that does it for you, you might find some of the bookwork in medicine rather dull and difficult to digest. Spend time thinking about practical applications. If you are learning about dry biochemical pathways, read also about clinical presentations of patients with problems in those pathways. You can look for case studies or even patient videos online that are relevant to your learning. You will want to buy some clinical textbooks early, so that you can read around clinical features of diseases. When learning about the pathology of the cervix, have a read about cervical smears, about the diagnosis and treatment of cervical cancer, think about how what you are learning will affect the care you give to patients. You might ask a friendly gynaecologist if you can sit in on their colposcopy clinic. See as many patients as possible, and read about the conditions that you have seen – you will remember information much more clearly if you can link it in your memory to a patient you have seen.
- Many students are most highly motivated by exams. If this is you, then look up the exam structure early in the year – look at the objectives, plan how you will cover them. Use past questions to structure your learning and to test yourself, write your own, learn in a group and write tests for each other. The revision section of this book will appeal to you (Chapter 9), and also some of the study strategies in Chapter 2.
- Does 'knowing that you've done a good job' motivate you to learn more? For many of us, praise and reward are important. If it is a major driver for you, you might want to be pragmatic in some of your learning. If you are sitting in an asthma clinic next Thursday, then learn about the management of asthma before then. You will feel like you understand what's going on, you will ask sensible questions, and the clinician in clinic is likely to be impressed – this will motivate you to study more. This simple technique works exceptionally well!
- There are a few students who thrive on external pressure. They love teachers who intimidate students, whereas most of their peers tend to hide in threatening environments, they thrive in them. If this is you, then you might want to try and create situations that will drive you to learn. Agree deadlines with tutors or your peers, agree to teach students in your year or the year below; encourage them to try and catch you out, so that you know that you will have to learn your topic well.

Of course, you will not fit singly into any one of these five vignettes, but you will know which ones apply most to you. You are also likely to find that different topics might have different motivations for you. Clearly there will not be a single strategy that applies to you. You can't only read about the conditions that you have seen patients with or you will never learn about the rare ones. Similarly, if you are 100% exam focused, you might miss out on the things that are important but not examined. However, knowing and manipulating what motivates you in order to maximise your study is a key skill. It might even be worth putting a Post-it up on the wall above your desk, reminding you of what motivates you.

Self-regulation of study skills

Students who are aware of how they are learning (this is called metacognition) tend to perform much better than those who don't. This book is largely about helping you develop effective study skills, and an awareness of when and how to use which ones. How aware of your learning are you? How consciously do you make choices in how you learn? Did you use different methods to learn different topics at school? If not, why not? The more you can learn to think about *how* you are learning, the more you will develop as an effective learner.

EXERCISE

Think about the following tasks. Spend 2 minutes on each task thinking about how you would go about it. Time yourself; it will be time well spent.
- You have a list of complications of diabetes to learn.
- You have to memorise a list of drug names for treating high blood pressure; the names all sound rather foreign to you.
- You have to learn the surface markings of the various lobes of the lungs so that you know which one is where when you are examining a patient.
- You have to learn how to take blood.

How easy was it to plan how you would go about each task? Was your plan for each task different, or the same? Did you have several options for each task, or just one? The more options and the more active your decisions, the easier you will find learning. If you tended to think of just one method of learning ('I'd just keep repeating it until I remembered' or 'I'd just learn it'), then you are likely to benefit from spending extra time on pp. 27–36 of Chapter 2, and it might be worthwhile finding out if there are some study skills workshops run by your university. Improving in your study skills is an investment that will really pay off.

Learning how to learn was the most important thing I got from medical school, unfortunately I didn't realise this until the second year!

Rebecca, finalist

How do you know that you know enough?

The A-level syllabus that you studied was well defined, in terms of both breadth of topics and depth that you need to go to in each topic. This is not so true at medical school and, as we have already mentioned, knowing when to stop can be a challenge. Some students are excellent at monitoring their progress, and use the sort of tricks that we discuss in the chapter on learning knowledge (Chapter 2), but others either tend to learn far too much (and run out of time) or learn far too little.

EXERCISE

Think for a minute how you know when you have learnt enough on a topic. What evidence do you use that you know something?

This evidence that you rely on to know that you know enough on a topic may be objective, subjective or 'non-evidence'. **Objective measures** might include testing yourself from a book of past questions, or writing questions before you start learning from the course objectives and seeing if you can answer them when you think you have finished learning; perhaps you try and explain it to someone else and see if you can answer all their questions. More **subjective evidence** will include others telling you that you are knowledge-able, or perhaps you make a judgement that you can now understand something that previously you found rather complex, perhaps you look at the learning objectives and make a judgement on whether you have covered them. **Non-evidence** tends to be pretty useless, it includes judgements such as judging the number of hours that you have looked at a page, or how many books you have on the subject, or how tidy your notes look as some 'guesstimate' of how much you have learnt.

You are likely to use a blend of these three approaches, and students who tend to cross-reference objective and subjective measures are likely to have a far more accurate idea of where they are up to in their learning. Students who use non-evidence tend to be rather surprised when they fail exams – 'but I spent hours looking at the books' or 'but my notes are always so perfect'.

Conception of learning

What is learning for? What is learning about? Do you see learning as a passive increase in knowledge, or perhaps as memorisation of facts; perhaps you see learning as a way of gaining information that you can apply in practice, or perhaps you learn in order to try and make sense of the world around you. Students who tend to try and make personal meaning out of what they learn seem to be more motivated and achieve deeper learning.

You might have left secondary school thinking that learning was about getting facts into your head. If so, you should be aware of the transition in higher education, where you will be expected to question, debate, weigh up different, conflicting evidence in order to try and make some sort of sense of the information in front of you and how it relates to the world around you. You can speed that transition by questioning yourself: asking 'What if . . . ?' or 'Why . . . ?' and 'What use is this information?'.

As an example, when you are learning about diabetes, you might ask yourself 'What if diabetes was not a disease that either you had or you didn't have, but a continuum between normal blood sugar and damagingly high blood sugar?' Perhaps you will ask 'why is the threshold for diagnosing diabetes a fasting sugar of 7.0 mmol/L and not 7.4 mmol/L?' If you have a very concrete idea of facts, valid questions like these might be uncomfortable, it's better to have this discomfort early on, and learn to manage it than later in your career. You might have to trust us on this one!

Learning in groups

Collaborative learning has its pros and cons. Some students feel that they can only really learn through discussion and debate with others, and they tend to struggle to find people with whom you can discuss everything that you have learnt. If this is you, you will benefit from reading the chapters on study skills (Chapter 2) and revision (Chapter 9). In contrast, some students find that they hate to study with others. These students tend to struggle to know whether they are learning to the right depth, and they really struggle with clinical and communication skills learning, as feedback from peers and peer practice is crucial. If you fit into this group, the chapters on clinical and communication skills learning (Chapters 3 and 4) and working in a group (Chapter 5) will be particularly relevant to you.

Mood

Mood affects learning. Have you ever been so angry or frustrated that you were unable to study? Or so passionate about a subject that everything you read seemed to make sense? 'Feeling' can be intimately involved with 'thinking'?

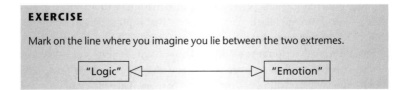

EXERCISE

Mark on the line where you imagine you lie between the two extremes.

"Logic" ◁──────────────▷ "Emotion"

Are there things that particularly swing you one way or another along this line? Some people find certain triggers throw them into emotional responses; guilt, for example, drives some to study but handicaps others. How about anxiety? Do you spend too much time worrying about the things you haven't done rather than getting on and doing them?

What if you are on the other end of the scale, emotion never affects your thinking and learning, would you be missing out on the passion, the buzz of knowing that you are 'on a roll'? How will you develop empathy if you can't see how emotion affects people's decisions (logically, surely everyone should agree to take part in medical research)? What about teamwork skills – how will you relate to others if you can't see the emotional contexts in which they exist?

Think about where you are on the line, and consider at what point on that line you might be more productive. Spend some time considering how you can actively manage the triggers and swings to be a little more productive a little more of the time. We have worked with many students, and the simplest strategies are usually the best – a young woman whose studying used to be distracted by regular family crises that she would worry about moved out of home. When phone calls replaced knocks on her bedroom door, she discovered that she could switch off her phone while she was studying, and she could study with a clear head.

Sometimes emotion clouds *all* your thoughts, and that's a time to get help. Indeed, everyone will struggle with the way that they are feeling, and the way that that affects their work at one time or another in their careers. In Chapter 8 we talk about avenues to ensure that you gain support when you need it.

VARK: using your senses

Think about incense. What comes immediately to mind? For some people they will see something relating to incense – perhaps the smoke curling up from a burning pot. Others will hear something – perhaps the ringing noise that an incense burner in church makes when it is swung, or the word incense being said. Others might see the word as it is written, perhaps think about the different meanings of the word: 'pieces of fragrant substance' or 'to infuriate'. Finally, you might think about the movements that you would make to light or to swing the incense around.

It seems that some people have a visual preference, others an auditory or aural preference. Some prefer to read or write things to learn them, and others have a strong kinesthetic preference – that is physically to do things. The VARK learning style has come up for criticism, but it has some uses. Look at the following descriptions and think of how much they each apply to you.

Visual people will like to use colour and shapes, they draw flowcharts and like to have everything in sight in front of them. They like books that are visually appealing, with small blocks of text, plenty of tables and diagrams. They might find learning visual topics like anatomy much easier than memorising lists of words.

Aural people like to listen, they think lectures are better than books, and like it when someone explains things to them in words, or they explain to others. They remember the anecdotes from the lecture, or what that patient said, and sometimes they forget to write things down as they are too busy listening. They are not fond of books, and tend to read books by forming the words in their heads. Sometimes their lips move when they are reading.

Those with a **read/write preference** tend to like books and texts and lists. They might copy out chunks of text from the book to form their notes, which are often quite lengthy and quite dry. They are good at spelling and can remember lists of words. They might look at a foreign word and work out what it means from similar words that they know.

Kinaesthetic learners like to learn by doing. They like practical applications – 'this goes there'. Real-life examples are great, and learning by trial and error really consolidates their learning. Abstract things are more difficult for them, and they strive to think of applications for what they are learning.

EXERCISE

For each of these preferences rate whether you think you are strong (you often think and learn in this way), average (you sometimes think and learn in this way) or weak (you rarely think or learn in this way)

	Weak	Average	Strong
Visual learning			
Aural/auditory learning			
Read/write learning			
Kinaesthetic learning			

Most people have a preference: some have strong preferences, others have a more even spread.

Think about your preferences, your strengths. This will give some indication of the sorts of tasks and subjects that you will find easiest. Think about how you can capitalise on your strengths:

- If you are a visual person, are you making best use of colour, of pictures? Would you be better making your notes on a pad of A3 rather than A4 so that you can see more in one glance? Do you take one of those four- or 10-colour pens into lectures with you? If not, why not? Do you try and convert difficult concepts into flow charts or cartoons? You will like the section on concept mapping in Chapter 2.

- If you are an auditory person, then do you make the best use of lectures, sitting near the front, away from distractions? Have you tried using tapes or reading your notes out loud? Do you ever put difficult facts to music to help you remember? You will find teaching and explaining to others really useful. How about starting a study group, or a debating society?
- If you like the written word, you can write brief descriptions of diagrams or flowcharts. You can change the words that your notes are written in, choosing your own words, so that you are sure that you are processing the information. You can write down patient stories, make lists and write essays. You might well like studying in libraries. Perhaps you could start an online group with others from your medical school or other medical schools where you explain things to each other on a messageboard or wiki.
- If you have a kinaesthetic approach, you will want to find practical applications for what you are learning. Get out there and do things – if you have seen a patient with a diabetic foot ulcer you will find it much easier to read about it. Apply what you have learned whenever you can, search for relevance. Use your imagination and imagine things happening when you read about them.

Think also about your weaknesses and how you can address them. There are two main approaches here. First you can try and redesign the task to play to your preferences. If you have to memorise a list of drug names and you are terrible at read/write but strong on auditory memory, make up a song or a poem and sing it out loud. If you have a preference for visual things, turn the words into pictures: the drug zopiclone might become a number of identical (clones) Z-shaped floppy aliens (zoppy), all sleepy in bed (zopiclone is a sleeping pill).

The second way that you might address your weaknesses is to train yourself to be stronger in these areas. Timetable extra time for the tasks that you might find challenging, and ask your peers what tricks they use. You can find others with similar preferences to you (the incense exercise is a good one, although lots of people say 'the smell', which doesn't fit well into VARK, but is discussed more in Chapter 9) and find out how they learn. If, as a group, you all hate learning vocabulary then at least you can empathise when you are testing each other on drug names – you will most likely learn at a similar rate.

You can find out more about VARK at www.vark-learn.com, or by typing VARK into your favourite internet search engine. There is not a huge amount of evidence for VARK over any of the other dimensions of learning listed above but, like the others, it is useful to help you think about where your strengths and weaknesses lie, and how you can capitalise on your strengths and actively manage your weaknesses.

Learning styles

As we mentioned at the start of this chapter, different learning style inventories tend to measure different combinations of the aspects of learning that we have listed. If your medical school has a progressive curriculum, you might well fill out a questionnaire on your learning style, and even get some numbers or a graph that will summarise your preferences. We would recommend that you look through this chapter a couple of times, and actually do the exercises and answer the questions. Write some notes on where you identify your strengths and weaknesses, triggers that upset your learning, and tips that maximise your learning.

Summary

This chapter has asked you to make multiple judgements about factors that affect your learning, which is not something you might have done before. Your judgements might not have been terribly accurate, and we would recommend that you revisit this chapter again when you have read the remainder of the book and had a chance to think in more depth about what factors affect your learning.

The multiple aspects within this chapter have made it rather complex. You might find Figure 1.1 useful in summarising the chapter – you can mark on

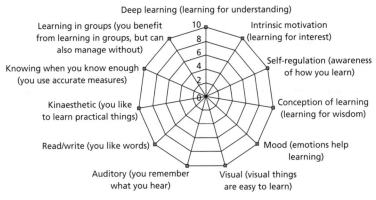

Figure 1.1 Summary.

each axis where you think your strengths are (perhaps you decide 10 relates to strength, or no problem).

References and further reading

Coffield, F. (2004). *Learning styles and pedagogy in post-16 learning: a systematic and critical review*. London, Learning and Skills Research Centre.
Coffield, F. (2004). *Should we be using learning styles?: what research has to say to practice*. London, Learning and Skills Research Centre.

Questions and answers

Q: I have done an online test for VARK, and my kinaesthetic score is low – will I have trouble learning clinical skills?

A: The predictive validity of these different tests is not great. Some studies have suggested that students with either deep (learn to remember and understand) or pragmatic (learn to pass exams effectively) learning styles do better in medical school exams than those with superficial styles (cram facts for the exams, skim over the top), but this really isn't rocket science to understand. The usefulness in these inventories is that they encourage you to think about your preferences and the way that you tend to learn – do you think that this judgement is true for you? If you tend to avoid practising when learning a skill, how are you going to make sure that you practise your clinical skills a great deal when you are learning them? See Chapter 3 for an in-depth description of effective clinical skills learning.

Q: My medical school not only makes me do learning style inventories, but also inventories on how I work in a team – it drives me mad!

A: There are inventories for almost everything you can imagine, as a significant proportion of the world is made up of people who like to measure things, everything; in fact they even make up new things in order to measure them. As you might guess from this chapter, our emphasis is less on formal, accurate, statistically significant measurement, but much more on using these tools pragmatically in order to develop your self-awareness. We know that students who develop self-awareness with respect to learning outperform their peers, so see what you can take out from the exercises. Perhaps you want to find Professor Coffield's papers (which critiques learning styles in depth) (mentioned in Chapter 2) and engage in a discussion with your course convenor.

Chapter 2 **Learning knowledge**

OVERVIEW

This chapter introduces some of the key issues and strategies for learning knowledge. We discuss the different types of knowledge and tips for improving your learning based on what we know about how memory works. Finally we discuss different learning environments and how to make best use of them.

Introduction

There is one thing that we can be pretty sure about – that you are intelligent. You did well at school (you might even have been near the top of the class) and some of you will have relied on a good memory, but not a great deal of study, to pass your exams. Unfortunately, medical school is not like secondary school. The curriculum is not as clearly set as for A-levels, and it has a tendency to change a little while you are still trying to follow it. The volume of work is huge, too big for even the best minds to hold without effort, and too much information to cram into your head the week before the exam. The source of knowledge might be different too: you might have been told what to learn at school – learn the classes and do the set homework and you will do well at most secondary schools. In medicine you will not get taught everything that you need to know, and yet you will still be expected to learn it – to work out what you need to learn, to work out ways of learning it, to work out ways of knowing when you have learnt it, and to get on and learn it.

This drastic change of emphasis comes as a culture shock to many. This chapter highlights some of the issues with learning in medical school, and looks to established theories from educational psychology and established

How to Succeed at Medical School: an essential guide to learning. By Dason Evans and Jo Brown. Published 2009 by Blackwell Publishing, ISBN: 978-1-4051-5139-9.

study skills techniques to make your learning as efficient and effective as possible.

There are some key messages running through this chapter, which might be worth highlighting here.

- Learning to learn effectively and efficiently, like any other skill, requires deliberate and reflective effort over time. If you want to learn a new way of learning, it will take 3 months or so of practice before you become fluent. If you invest time and effort now, these skills will stay with you and help you for the rest of your life.
- There is no end to what you *could* learn in medicine, so you will need to learn what is important, and when you can tell you know enough about a subject.
- The only way to survive the load of learning at medical school is through regular, active, self-directed learning. It is probably possible to pass the exams in the first 2 years of most curricula by cramming if you have a good memory, but it won't be possible after this, and your knowledge will be seriously deficient. Start studying for being a doctor from week 1 of your course.
- Spend time not only thinking about *what* you are learning, but also *how* you are learning – what works for you? What works for this task? How could you improve your learning?
- Learning in medicine is a lifelong process, medical school is just the start, you might as well try and get the foundations right.

How do I know what to learn?

Medical education is unlike other types of higher education. Medicine has no start and no end, and it is close to impossible to define exactly the knowledge, skills and attitudes that are required to be a doctor. Medicine is rapidly changing, so by the time you get to the end of a 4-, 5- or 6-year curriculum, exactly what you need to be able to know and to be able to do, will have changed. Understandably, students struggle and stress trying to find out what they are expected to know, and this section aims to give some pointers on how to find out. The bad news is that there isn't one published list of what is needed to make a good doctor, but the good news is that there are plenty of pointers out there. You'll need to make some judgements about what you want and need to learn, but for the rest of your professional life you'll need to make those judgements, so it's not a bad habit to get into.

Your medical school is likely to publish a curriculum listing core required knowledge in one form or another (perhaps as a list of core conditions), and this should provide you with some guidance. It might change, and more importantly it might not reflect what you need to know to be a safe and effective doctor, so you will need to spend some time considering what else you should know and to what depth. Textbooks are handy, looking through the table of contents of a medium-sized core text will give you a good idea, as will looking through the index of some thin undergraduate books. You might want to look at both clinical books and basic science books (anatomy, pathology, physiology etc.), as you will be expected to learn hard science and its clinical application.

Self-directed versus teacher-directed learning

In some secondary schools the teaching is excellent. You were taught what you needed to know to do well in your exams. Learn your lessons, do your set-work well and you did well in your GCSEs and in your A-levels. Medicine (and indeed most higher education) is different. You will need to learn to take control of your own learning; after all, this is how you will be learning for the rest of your professional life as a doctor. Keep a notebook or a section of your diary where you can jot down things you want to look up, and set aside regular time to do so. These might be things that you think are important for exams or for your practice as a doctor, or they might be things that you find interesting and might make you a more rounded doctor.

Just learning the taught components of your course and doing the set assignments will not be enough to become a good doctor.

> *I prefer to be taught things, and have always gone to teachers to find things out. It was a real culture shock at my medical school when they just replied 'how are you going to look that up?' Sometimes I wish they would just teach me.*
>
> Catriona, first-year medical student.

Binge learning versus regular learning

There is no way of escaping it, you will need to develop a habit of regular self-directed learning. Our Chapter 8 on life–work balance covers this in more depth. You might in the past have crammed for exams, and your memory might be such that you can memorise a whole lot of facts and hold them in your memory for a week or two. There are three problems with doing this in medicine. First, the volume of facts will become too great to hold; at some point you will not be able to manage, and at that point you will realise that you are actually years behind in your knowledge. Second, you will not be asked to just regurgitate facts, instead you will be asked to apply knowledge: you need a deep level of understanding to be able to do this, and cramming doesn't give you that kind of level.

Finally, and most importantly, you are not studying to pass exams, you are studying to be a doctor. Cramming information in your head just before an exam and forgetting it shortly after will not help you care for patients, regardless of whether you passed.

You will need a diary, and a timetable, and you will need to plan regular self-directed learning, some of which will involve looking up new topics, and some of which will involve reviewing your previous learning to consolidate it into long-term memory (more on this later in the chapter). If you get into good habits early in the course, they will pay major dividends during the course and long after.

Lifelong learning and Continuing Professional Development

The phrase lifelong learning is a bit of a mantra in higher education, and gets brought out at every opportunity. Skipping all the rhetoric, as a doctor you need to continue learning, all the time, day in day out for the rest of your professional life. For the vast majority of the time, no-one will tell you what you need to learn. You will need to know what you do know (relatively easy), know what you don't know (which is harder), prioritise what you need to know, or what you might need to know (difficult if you have a tendency to be indecisive), work out a way of learning it (bad news, plenty of studies show that exotic conferences are a terrible way of learning), and work out a way of knowing when you know enough on that topic and can move on (Figure 2.1). Appraisals, some curricula, your mentors and drug reps touting their wares might all help you, but the emphasis will always come down to you.

One of your aims at medical school has to be to learn how to learn, and learn how to continue to learn, to keep up to date. It is daunting, but actually it's fun too.

Depth versus breadth

Here is a key issue that students struggle with. One student we worked with had a tendency to always study to far too great a depth. She was working with a group of others close to finals and they agreed to go away and study liver disease over the next 2 days and then come back and test each other. This student became lost in the molecular pathology of primary biliary cirrhosis, finding deeper and deeper books to go into, and never got to read about gallstones. It would be possible to study for a PhD on the molecular pathology of this rare condition, and still not understand it completely. As a doctor, it is not a condition that you are likely to see often (if at all), let alone need to know the molecular pathology of it. On the flip side of the coin, we have also seen plenty of students who do the opposite: they buy the thinnest books possible and can write two lines on any condition in medicine – only two lines though! (Figure 2.2).

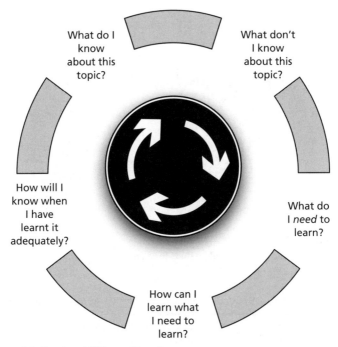

Figure 2.1 Planning Self-Directed Learning.

Working out to what depth you need to learn is a difficult balancing act. You cannot and will not ever know everything, and yet you probably want to know more than the minimum. Throughout the rest of this chapter we try and give tips on different ways you might check that you are working to an appropriate depth.

> *I really like to understand things fully. Sometimes I spend hours and hours on one small thing, looking in the library and on the net to try and understand it completely. I ran out of time in my revision and did badly in my first year exams – I think I've learnt my lesson.*
>
> Dimitris, second-year medical student

One answer: Bloom's taxonomy

Benjamin Bloom made a name for himself leading a group of educational psychologists in an attempt to define different levels of knowledge, in order to guide students and their examiners. He defined seven levels of knowledge, which are often used religiously by educationalists (Table 2.1). As with any

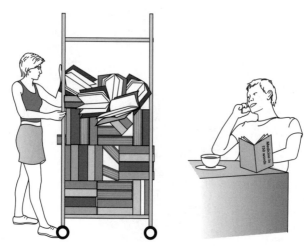

Figure 2.2 Finding the right depth to study to can be difficult.

Table 2.1 Bloom's levels of knowledge (adapted from Bruning, Schraw et al. 2004).

Knowledge (remember)	You know enough to be able to recite knowledge by rote (for example, you can recite the 15 causes of clubbing)
Comprehension (understand)	You understand the knowledge, so can explain it to others (for example, you can explain what clubbing is)
Application (apply)	You can use the knowledge you have to solve problems (you use your knowledge of clubbing to try and work out why the patient in front of you has clubbed fingers)
Analysis (analyse)	You can use the knowledge you have to compare and contrast with other knowledge and see how it fits in with other people's assumptions and/or hypotheses (for examples, compare and contrast type 1 and type 2 diabetes; compare and contrast the electron as a particle and the electron as an electromagnetic wave)
Synthesis (create)	You can use knowledge, integrated with other knowledge, to produce new hypotheses (for example, you know glucose crosses the placenta, and that insulin does not; you know that in diabetes glucose tends to run high, so you hypothesise that the baby of a woman with diabetes will produce high levels of insulin itself, and so will be at risk of going 'hypo' after birth)
Evaluation (evaluate)	You use your knowledge to assess, critique or judge others

model, it isn't perfect, but it is particularly useful to help you think about the purpose and the depth of knowledge that you are learning.

At medical school you will be expected to learn knowledge at more than a basic level. You will be asked to apply your knowledge, use it to problem solve, use it to critique papers and use it to hypothesise and create new ideas – simply knowing and understanding will not be enough.

Imagine that you are seeing a person with diabetes who has quite poor blood glucose control. Being able to recite a memorised list of causes for poor diabetic control is not going to help you very much – you will need to be able to take that knowledge, apply it, investigate what is going on for the patient, hypothesise which causes are most likely, test those hypotheses one way or another, and explain it all to the patient. Most of your exams will try and test these higher levels of knowledge, and when studying you should use techniques to ensure that you are learning knowledge to this level, more of this comes later.

EXERCISE

Look at the following exam questions; to what level of Bloom's taxonomy do they assess knowledge?

Q1 The following are causes of clubbing (true or false)

Q2 A man presents with clubbing and jaundice, which of the following are likely diagnoses?

Q3 A man presents with clubbing and shortness of breath, which one of the following investigations would be most appropriate?

Q4 Critique the box (Figure 2.3) 'what is clubbing?', and use your knowledge to suggest improvements.

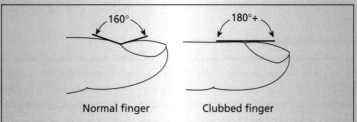

Figure 2.3 What is clubbing? Clubbing is a physical sign, a favourite of clinicians, where the bed of the nail is swollen, so that the finger nail or toe nail, rather than sliding downwards into the digit looks like it slopes in the opposite direction.

The mind, memory and learning

Without wishing to upset all those neurophysiologists and neuropsychologists, no-one really seems to understand how memory works. There are a couple of theories though, borne out by experimental research, which do provide some pointers on how memory might work particularly on how to maximise learning.

Left brain, right brain

Positron emission tomography (PET) scans and functional magnetic resonance imaging (MRI) scans as well as older electrophysiology work show that if you are right-handed, the left-hand side of your brain seems to relate to words, fact, logic, whereas the right-hand side deals much more with emotion, feelings and imagery. The theory goes that if you use both halves of your brain while learning, you are more likely to remember. This seems true: if you use as many senses and exaggeration and emotion when trying to learn something, you are more likely to remember it. One of the causes of clubbing is pus in the lungs (which occurs when there are lung abscesses, and conditions called empyema and bronchiectasis). If you visualise someone with hugely clubbed fingers, imagine pus dripping out from their lungs through their chest wall, dripping on the floor. It makes you feel sick, it is green and smelly, your imaginary person uses his or her clubbed finger nails to pick at the pus. Spend a moment imagining this (look up a picture of clubbing if needs be), run through all your senses and exaggerate them (what can you hear, smell, feel, taste, see?) and do the same with your emotions (perhaps you are afraid, or disgusted, you feel nauseous and so forth). If you hold this image in your head and revisit it once or twice, you will never forget pus in the lung as a cause of clubbing.

> *I really love using colour and pictures, I remember things so much better when I can see them.*
>
> Sian, third-year medical student

The vaccination model of memory

As a health care professional, you will be vaccinated against hepatitis B. You will be given the first injection, and this will cause a minor immune reaction, your antibodies will rise, and then fall. When given a second injection, your immune memory will be heightened, the same with the third. So with each injection your immune response and immune memory is strengthened. Not only are several injections better than one injection for strength and longevity of immune memory, but the timing also seems important – one injection today and the second in 5 years' time, is likely to be pretty useless.

There are parallels with memory, of course. If you learn a list of causes of clubbing, and don't look at it for a year, you will be lucky if you can remember it. If you learn it now, review it in 3 days', 3 weeks' and 3 months' time, you will probably remember it for life (the rule of three's). This is one of the reasons why most medical schools have exams frequently, and each exam will often cover the content of the last exam, in addition to the learning you have done since then. This is to encourage you to revisit and review your learning on a regular basis.

This has some practical implications for studying. Use your diary or timetable (see Chapter 8) to mark down review sessions – perhaps one evening a week. Use this time to review notes that you made this week, 3 weeks ago and 3 months ago. If you use active learning principles (see later), you will be able to review your notes quickly and efficiently and extend your memory of the topics far beyond your peers.

Semantic networks

One of the leading models of memory is that memories are encoded in networks. One item of knowledge is linked to other items of knowledge like some massive, messy spider's web, with knowledge sitting at intersections of the silk, and the web representing the links. Clubbing links to what you know about the anatomy of the fingers, links to the possible diagnoses, each of which links to what you know about them. There is also probably now a link to a revolting image of pus.

Memory is, therefore, constructed by linking new learning with your prior knowledge (interestingly enough, even if your prior knowledge on the subject is rather poor), and the strength of a memory, or of learning, depends on the strength of those links. In turn, the strength of those links depends on how many times you use them.

As an example, another cause of clubbing is inflammatory bowel disease, particularly two conditions called Crohn's disease and ulcerative colitis. You could try and learn that as an isolated fact, or you could link it in with what you know of bowel diseases. If when you learn about causes of diarrhoea (such as Crohn's disease and ulcerative colitis) you think about the features you will look for on examination (such as clubbing), and when you read about the anatomy and histopathology of the bowel you consider systemic manifestations of bowel disease (such as, you guessed it, clubbing), then that link between clubbing and inflammatory bowel diseases will be much stronger, and if you see a patient with clubbing, bowel disease will spring into your mind, similarly if you see a patient with Crohn's disease, you will know to look for clubbing.

The relevance for your learning is that when learning new things, always try and build links with what you know already, this will strengthen both the new learning and your prior knowledge.

Active learning, passive learning

Have you ever seen someone asleep over (or under) a book? I have a fantastic picture of my brother asleep on the sofa with a copy of the *British National Formulary* covering his eyes. We labelled it 'learning by osmosis'. Thinking about yourself, have you ever sat and stared at a page, read the same paragraph over and over before you realised that you hadn't taken in a word of it? We have seen plenty of students who sit and read books, look at the words, often spending many hours doing so, but then still don't seem to do well in the exams.

Effective learning is an active process requiring effort and energy. The volume of learning required in medicine is so much that even those with outstanding memories will not be able to just soak it all up, and this will be a shock for many. Similarly, the fact that you will need to apply knowledge, will mean that those who try and just learn flat facts, to recall a paragraph or two of a core text, will have a lot of trouble taking that knowledge and using it in other contexts.

Tips for active learning

Before learning

- Ask questions – Why am I learning this? What will it tell me? How will I know when I have learnt it?
- Obtain an overview (look perhaps at the headings and subheadings in a text book)
- Write down what you know already on some rough paper, perhaps as a brainstorm or concept map (see later in the chapter)
- Write down some key questions that you should be able to answer at the end of your learning – perhaps use past exam questions.

During learning

- Don't write things down word for word, rather listen or read a section, and then write down what you think you need to know, in your own words
- Write notes reliant on key words (see below)
- See where your learning links in with other things you know. Look at your brainstorm/concept map – is it right, what can you add to it?

After learning

- Tidy up your notes
- Has your learning told you what you needed?
- Rewrite your network of key information
- Can you put your notes away and answer those questions that you identified at the start?
- Can you explain what you leant to someone else? Here is a great role for a study group.

There are some tricks to making learning active; these principally revolve around the concept of **learning by doing**. Making notes is an example, and making notes in such a way that when you come to review them you will do more than just read them is a particularly useful technique, which will be discussed in the next few sections. Whatever method you use, think about your learning and ensure that it is active learning.

Making notes

The key principle: keywords

Just about all effective note taking, whether from books or lectures, whether conventional or more modern approaches, depends on the concept of 'keywords'. A keyword is a word or short phrase that sums up a sentence or an idea. The keyword itself should remind you of the content of that sentence or idea, and so keywords are personal – your keywords may not be the same as mine, depending on our different prior knowledge, although usually there is common ground. Keywords give enough information to trigger recall. This paragraph can be summarised with the four keywords (OK, key phrases) represented in Figure 2.4.

If you look at these keywords after reading the paragraph above, you should be able to recall what it was about. I haven't included 'word or short phrase' as I know that about keywords already. Notice that if you hadn't read that paragraph, the keywords might not be that useful ('personal' could mean any number of things), so keywords aid recall of something that you have read or heard, but are not that useful as a starting point. Books of lists are popular with medical students, and these are basically someone else's lists of keywords. Trying to memorise these lists really doesn't help learning, despite whatever the introduction to the book says!

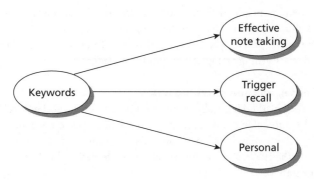

Figure 2.4 Key phrases.

Where keywords come into their strength is when you have made them yourself. You can summarise and remind yourself of huge chunks of text books or lectures with one or two keywords, and when revising and reviewing your notes these prompts should help you recall the main points. If they don't, you will need to glance at the book or lecture slides and you will very quickly say 'ah yes'.

If you are new to keywords, learning to make them can be quite difficult. You will need to practise and to review how you are progressing on a regular basis. Start with texts and lectures that are not too heavy on facts and figures – clearly trying to make keywords from a book of lists would not be a good start. Try and summarise a chapter of this book with keywords, and then after a day, see if the keywords remind you enough of the content for you to explain it to someone else. Go back to the keywords that didn't help, and see if you need them, of if you can rephrase them to work better for you. With a little practice, making keywords becomes second nature. For a book like this, a keyword or two for each paragraph is probably about right. This paragraph might be summarised by 'easy with deliberate practice', which reminds me not only that it is easy with practice, but that also practice is required, and 'deliberate practice' to me means practice where I think about how I am learning while I practise.

SQ3R

The SQ3R is quite time-consuming if you do it properly, and may be challenging if you have a high workload, but it does gives some good general principles for all note taking: – First **survey** the topic – have a look at reading lists, past exam papers, perhaps look at subheadings in a text book. Next **question** – why are you reading this? What do you want to get out of it? How will you know when you know enough? **Read** to understand, a paragraph at a time, without making notes. Next **re-read** to take notes, and finally **review** whether the notes do the job.

The useful principles with this model are that reading around a subject and actively thinking about what your learning needs to give you will make your learning active, provide you structure in your learning, and should help you to build new learning on top of your prior knowledge.

The Cornell method of taking notes

The Cornell method is a really simple modification of classical note taking to make the note taking and subsequent reviewing of those notes into active learning. It was developed by Walter Pauk (from Cornell University, of course) in the 1950s, and it is now widely used internationally. The secret is in the preparation.

Before you start making notes, before the lecture or before you sit down with a book, take your blank paper and draw three lines. Draw a line across the top of the page so that you have dedicated space for a title (date, topic, other such info.), draw a line across the page separating the bottom quarter – you will use this as a summary later, and finally draw a line down the left-hand side, about 5 cm (2 inches) from the left. Write your notes in the main body of the page (the right-hand side).

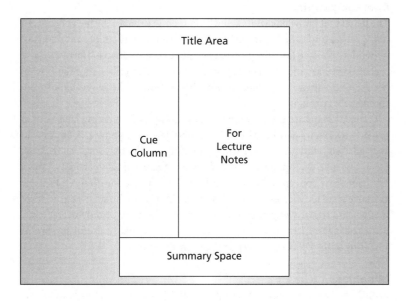

After the lecture, or when you close the book, look through your notes and tidy them up. Then on the left-hand column, write in the key words or prompts or summary points that will help you recall the notes that you took. Finally, at the bottom of the page, write a one-sentence summary of what the page is all about.

This method is particularly useful in two respects. First it makes you review your notes and makes sure you understand them. The reviewing, summarising and bringing out key concepts makes your learning active. The second thing it enables is easy, active revision. When revising just cover up the right-hand side of the notes with a piece of rough paper – look at each summary point on the left and write on the rough paper the details that link to that point. When you have done that for all the summary points, check your rough paper against the underlying notes, what is missing?

Of course, you can adapt the Cornell method to the task at hand and to your preferred learning. Perhaps you can use the summary space to write a handful of short answer questions, then when revising you can give them a go without looking at the notes, then look at the summary points in the cue column – do you want to add anything to your answers? Then look at the notes on the right – what did you leave out?

Concept mapping

The belief that knowledge is linked within memory makes the idea of concept maps rather appealing. Concept maps are diagrammatic representations of networks of related knowledge. Each node in a concept map is a keyword, and each linkage has a direction and an annotation that described the relationship between keywords. A concept map of this section so far might look something like Figure 2.5.

Concept maps are useful when there are complex interacting facts, and to provide overviews of otherwise rather murky terrain. I know academics who keep all their references for academic papers in concept maps, so that they can see at a glance what papers to look for when researching a particular topic. You can draw concept maps by hand, or use software for doing it. Generic software such as Microsoft PowerPoint and Word can build simple concept maps using the drawing and connector tools; there are also dedicated software packages. Electronic concept maps are particularly useful for brainstorming as they allow you to rearrange concepts easily.

MindMaps

MindMaps, a term coined by Tony Buzan (1995), are a type of hierarchical concept map that makes use of colour and imagery (that right-brain–left-brain idea). They use keywords in a tree-like structure, and encourage the writer to use as much of their imagination as possible. Figure 2.6 shows you one of two MindMaps I have written on note taking, the actual content is not important, but you can see the use of imagery (corn for Cornell, keys for keywords, etc.) that helps me remember the different areas and their content.

The main challenge in making MindMaps is that it is difficult to guess where to place the main stems – often you will find that you didn't leave enough space for one or two of the sections. When making MindMaps from books, the general structure is reasonable to guess in advance from the subheadings and size of the various subsections. In lectures this is more tricky, although at the start of the presentation the lecturer might well give some structure ('Today I am going to cover three main aspects of diabetes'). Make

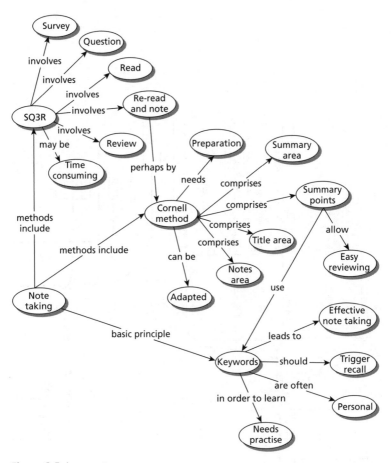

Figure 2.5 A concept map.

your MindMap on A3 and don't get too stressed if you have to go onto another piece of paper. Spend 10 minutes at the end of the lecture, or some other time that day in a spare moment to rewrite your MindMap as a best version – the rewriting will help it fit more logically to the page, and will help you review what you learnt. You might decide that you don't need everything that you wrote down, or that there is an area that looks a bit sparse and might need some additional bookwork to fill out.

MindMaps are personal things. They are best handwritten and annotated. Use colours and images that mean something to you. When revising, take a blank sheet of paper and see how much you can draw out again, then look at your original map and see what you missed. Use active techniques to revise,

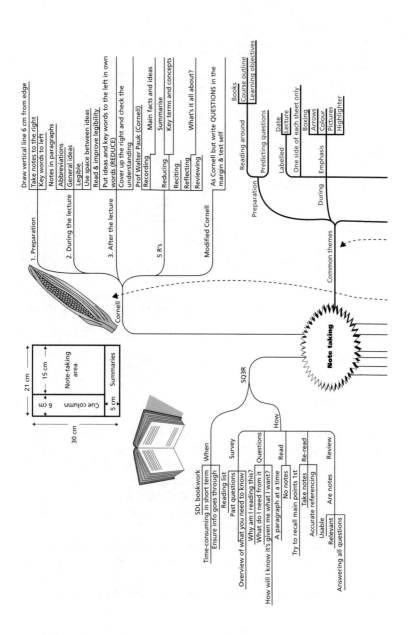

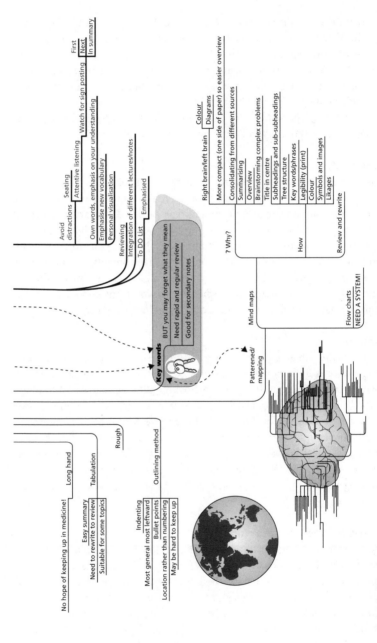

Figure 2.6 MindMaps.

there is too much on a complex MindMap for you to learn just by looking at it. Similarly there are books of MindMaps for medicine that you can buy. These are usually little more than lists arranged in a tree structure. The key benefits of MindMaps for learning are first that you learn by creating them, by colouring them, by thinking what images might help you remember, and second that they are personal to you.

Tony Buzan's book *Use Your Head* (1995) gives an excellent general guide to learning, and covers MindMaps in a lot more detail.

Cue cards

You can buy various size cue cards from most stationers. These are perfect if you tend to feel overloaded when revising. Make summary notes on to cue cards – one card one topic. Imagine a card on myocardial infarction: it could include key words summarising features on history, examination, special investigations, treatment, complications and pathology. You can carry it with you and try and remember what is on it in spare moments, and then check to see if you were right. You could do the same for many core conditions, and either review them in turn or, when you are confident, choose one at random. Perhaps ask a friend to select a card at random and test you.

Tables

Constructing tables is a fantastic way of summarising data. Let's think about respiratory examination: there are 20 or so steps to the examination, and 10 or so common clinical diagnoses, each with a different pattern of findings. Making a table with findings down one side and conditions across the top is great for highlighting the different findings between different conditions.

Making tables is very useful for summarising and understanding, but just looking at tables, perhaps in a book, is much less useful. Imagine the example above – it will have 200 bits of information in it – far too much to absorb by looking at it. If you want to revise a table, take a blank piece of paper and try and write it out again.

The right tools for the right job

You might be feeling frustration from this chapter – 'Hang on, which is the best way of making notes' – the answer is very much 'It depends!' The best way depends on the task in hand (both the complexity and the environment) and your personal preference. For some tasks Cornell will be the best option, for others a table might be best. If you are a visual person (see the section on learning styles, Chapter 1) then you might tend to have a preference for MindMaps, if you are more of a words person then you might lean more towards cue cards.

It is important to know that it takes up to 3 months to become slick at any new way of learning. If these concepts above are new to you, introduce them one at a time. Start with keywords, then when you are finding it easy to find the right keywords, perhaps try MindMaps or concept mapping for a couple of months. Keep a log of which methods seem to work for which tasks. Once you have mastered several methods, you will notice that you start using the most appropriate method automatically.

Learning environments

Learning from lectures

Some medical schools remain predominantly lecture based, whereas others use mostly small group work (see Chapter 5). All schools will use lectures at one time or another, and making the most out of them will help you a great deal.

Preparation is important, although many students find the organisation required challenging. Reading up on the topic before the lecture will help you understand the topic much more deeply. Imagine at the far extreme that you spent 20 minutes before the lecture making some notes on the topic of the lecture, using a leading text. You leave plenty of spaces in your notes, and anything that you don't understand after reading it twice, you just leave space. In the lecture you sit back and listen, annotate your notes and fill in the gaps. You can work from your notes (as opposed to the lecturer's handouts, which are likely not to be in your style) and concentrate on understanding. You could prepare the night before, or even get in a bit early and prepare over a coffee. Perhaps a more realistic alternative is that you spend 5 minutes the night before a lecture looking at the objectives of the lecture, and then just scribbling down the main subheadings from the relevant section of a text book. That way you might well trigger some prior knowledge, and in the lecture you will have a good idea of where the lecture is going.

> I used to think that just 'being there' was enough, only when I talked to some friends after a lecture did I realise that I hadn't picked up as much as them.
>
> Bruce, first-year medical student

During the lecture make sure that all your paper is labelled clearly with the lecture and the date – you will thank yourself 6 months later when you drop your file and paper goes everywhere! Think about where you want to sit in the lecture theatre. Aim to sit somewhere where you will have to concentrate, and where distractions will be at a minimum. If your friends tend to talk to you or distract you in other ways, save their company for the breaks, and sit away from them in lectures. If they object, tell them that you must be stupid or something because you really need to concentrate hard to understand lectures. Buy them a coffee and they will forgive you!

Pay particular attention to the lecturer signposting important points, or transitions between different parts of the lecture. Listen for 'importantly', 'don't forget', 'in summary', 'the (first, second, next . . .) key point that I want to make is . . .'

Write your notes in your own words, and use keywords and bullet points as appropriate. Concentrate on writing down *your understanding* rather than the words on the slides. Use emphasis in your notes – boxes and arrows, pictures and colours. Highlight key points and ensure that the headings are clear. Box or circle any new words and their definitions.

After the lecture, tidy up your notes, think about how this lecture fits in with other learning that you have had. You might even combine several different lecture notes if there is substantial overlap – the importance is that you can understand and apply what you have learnt, not that you can regurgitate one particular lecturer's presentation.

Once in a while you will have a terrible lecture. It will be all over the place, hard to follow and it will come with a handout that has had all headings removed to save space. You will be tempted to spend hours trying to make sense of it all – don't bother. Look at the objectives for the lecture (the school will have published them somewhere) and just open an appropriate book. Imagine the clinical lecture on infertility was impossible to follow – just open a book on gynaecology for general practice and look at the infertility section, it will give a good overview. When you understand the topic, if you really want to, then is the time to look back at the lecture. Hopefully this won't happen often, but it is important to be aware that if you are finding a lecture impossible to follow, it might not be your fault, and it might be a good indicator that you should use another source for your learning.

Learning from books

The same principles apply to learning from books as learning from lectures. Be attentive to your surroundings and possible distractions. If you are at home, turn the TV and radio off and put a do-not-disturb sign on the door. If you are working in the library, you might choose a seat that faces a wall to avoid watching the world go by.

It is probably best to make notes of one form or another, depending on the task in hand. Don't, whatever happens, just copy out chunks of text: unless you think about what you are reading, how will you learn it? Some people will just sit and read books, others annotate the pages (only if you own the book, please), but the trouble with that is that first the temptation is to think you are studying when you are, in fact, just looking at the page and, second, when you come to revise, you will have a whole mass of reading to do all over again. With deliberate, reflective practice, your notes should become a distillation of the key points, with an emphasis on the areas that you think are important, and that you, personally, think you might have difficulty remembering. In this way, your notes will be different from the books, and will be different from another student's notes on the same subject.

As discussed previously, making notes is not good enough on its own, they need to be useful notes, you need to review them at a regular basis, and when you review them you need to be learning actively (try to rewrite the key points, try to answer a couple of questions etc.).

Learning from the Internet

Here's an exercise: go to your favourite Internet search engine and type in 'George Bush is an alien' – if you use quotation marks it will only find that exact phrase. You will find plenty of evidence that its true, George Bush is an alien (apologies to Americans). Similarly 'HIV is not sexually transmitted' and 'radiation is good for you.' The Internet is therefore full of misinformation, interspersed with some high-quality information. Working out which category the information you find fits into can be challenging.

Every medical student should receive training on finding reliable information on the Internet. If you haven't, that is precisely the sort of request that will bring your medical librarian to tears of joy. There are some websites that give guidance on how to evaluate other websites for accuracy, one good one is www.quick.org.uk, which gives advice aimed at secondary schools, but is equally valid for the rest of us. Another, http://www.discern.org.uk/, gives a questionnaire specifically aimed at evaluating health-related websites.

You will find some **portals**, websites that act as gateways to other high-quality sites: www.doctors.org, the student BMJ and BMA learning are just three of many examples. Websites that have a clearly described peer review process are likely to provide more reliable information than others.

Finding that review article

The web does, of course, provide a quick way of identifying high-quality articles from peer-reviewed journals. Some of these articles may be of particular use to you, and these will include educational articles and review articles. Educational articles are those which are designed to refresh doctors and often provide great overviews on topics. The *BMJ*, for example, publishes a '10-minute consultation' series, and 'masterclass for GPs' series, and will provide you with a good overview of the clinical aspects, and especially clinical skills required for the diagnosis of a condition. Review articles review the published literature and provide an up-to-date summary of the current understanding of a disease, condition or treatment.

The principal free portal to search peer-reviewed journals is **PubMed**, which can be found at www.pubmed.org. It is worth playing with this website early in your studies at medical school, as an advanced understanding of how to use it will benefit you a great deal at all stages of your career. Particularly useful at your stage will be the 'Limits' tab – imagine that you are reading about headache. Putting 'headache' into the PubMed search field will retrieve over 40 000 articles, most of very little interest to you. Now use the 'Limits' tab and put in the following limits:

- articles published in the last year (so up to date)
- English language (unless you are bilingual)
- core clinical journals (you are not interested in pure research)
- under type of article click both 'Practice guideline' and 'Review'.

Now hit the 'go' button and you will be offered recent English language articles from the core clinical journals that review the literature or give guidelines for practice. Choose one or two of these and have a read!

If you use information from the article in an essay or your notes, make sure you **reference** it appropriately, more details about referencing and plagiarism can be found in Chapter 6, and your medical library will be able to give you further information, advice and training. It is worthwhile learning how to reference appropriately as soon as possible, as this is a skill that you will use throughout your career, and you can get into sticky water if you don't know the rules.

Summary

Learning knowledge is essential for a career in medicine. Learning is an active process that requires effort and engagement. Learning how to learn, just as with any other skill, needs practise (and plenty of it), experimentation and reflection. *Different sorts of knowledge* and *different sources of knowledge* may require different approaches to learning.

References and further reading

Buzan, T. (1995). *Use Your Head*. London, BBC.
Cottrell, S. (2003). *The Study Skills Handbook*. Basingstoke, Palgrave Macmillan.

Questions and answers

Q: How do I know when I know enough?

A: Buried in this chapter are a number of strategies – you can consult curricula, look at the contents of thin undergraduate books, practise past papers, write your own questions ('having read about diabetes, would I be able to explain it to a patient? Let me practise on a friend and see') and, perhaps most importantly, study with others in your year, and compare your depth and breadth of understanding with theirs. We discuss more on the pros and cons of collaborative learning in Chapter 5 (collaborative learning).

Q: What is the point of making notes when I never look at them again?

A: Exactly, you need to build time in to your schedule to review notes regularly. Think about the review when you are writing the notes and plan to make the reviewing as active as possible – perhaps by writing questions or setting tasks that if you can complete will tell you that you know the topic.

Q: My flatmate never does any work, and he does really well in his exams

A: Odds are that he studies harder than he admits. Perhaps he just crams for his exams, in which case he will not remember much of what he learnt once the exams are over – do you want him looking after your mother if he qualifies? Why not aim to work harder and become a better doctor. When he fails, he'll appreciate your support.

Q: Is this chapter saying that I need to study all the time?

A: Yes and no. You need to be prepared to study over and above the 9 to 5 of the working week. This is the reality of a career as a doctor, and if you just want a 9 to 5 job with great evenings and weekends, you need to take some careers advice. Clearly you need a good balance between study and recreation, and if you are studying all evening every evening, you are doing something wrong. We think that getting the balance right is so important that we have committed a whole chapter (Chapter 8) to the topic.

Q: Writing notes takes ages – wouldn't it be better just to read the book?

A: If you are just starting out making notes, it will take time and effort to improve in speed and accuracy. Think about the words and abbreviations that you use – are you making best use of keywords, headings, drawings? Review your notes – are they too detailed? Have you, perhaps, just copied out chunks of text because it is easier than thinking? Good notes will help you review and revise topics quickly and easily, and should guarantee active learning. Your university will run study skills workshops on how to make notes – if you continue to have trouble why not book into one?

Chapter 3 **Learning clinical skills**

OVERVIEW

This chapter covers how you can work out what you need to learn, it discusses clinical examination skills and practical skills – how to learn them from books, from simulation and with patients. The clinical learning environment is very different from the classroom environment. We'll give you some tips on how to make the most of your tutors, and how to make the most of the time when tutors are not around. Finally we will cover feedback – how to give effective feedback, how to get effective feedback and how to learn from the feedback that you are given.

Introduction

Clinical skills (along with clinical communication skills) are what make doctors. Without the ability to take a history and examine the patient you will not be able to make a diagnosis. Without practical skills such as cardiopulmonary resuscitation, taking blood, inserting drips, you will not be able to conduct further investigations and treatment. Without effective clinical **communication skills**, you will not be able to explain treatment options to the patient and enable them to understand and to choose the right option for them. You will start to learn these skills at medical school, and you'll continue to improve and learn for the rest of your professional life.

The next chapter specifically covers clinical communication skills – the evidence base for learning clinical communication skills, how to make the most from learning in simulation and how to improve your clinical communication skills in the clinical environment. There is a recurring theme in both these

How to Succeed at Medical School: an essential guide to learning. By Dason Evans and Jo Brown. Published 2009 by Blackwell Publishing, ISBN: 978-1-4051-5139-9.

chapters, and we make no apologies for highlighting it repeatedly: you cannot learn a skill without knowing how to do that skill, without practising it, and practising it a lot, and without receiving feedback. All three parts are important, but practising is the part which is most commonly neglected – compare with any other skill whether it be playing a violin or playing football – to become an expert, you need thousands of hours of deliberate, reflective practice.

Learning skills is different to learning knowledge, but needs just as much commitment to time and effort. To learn a skill you need to know how to do that skill (what each step is, why you do each step, and what your findings will mean), you need to practise deliberately, thoughtfully and endlessly, and you need to receive and act on plenty of appropriate feedback. If you cover these three aspects, you'll be set for life.

On first encounter, the clinical learning environment can be a daunting place. It is unstructured, often chaotic and requires a lot of self-directed learning. If you are seen to be keen and enthusiastic, and if you actively seek out learning opportunities, then people will go out of their way to teach you, and provide you with even more learning opportunities. You'll feel valued and learn lots more than your peers and you will be better prepared for being a junior doctor.

How do I know what to learn?

Finding out the sort of skills that you need to learn at medical school is slightly easier than what knowledge you need to know (see Chapter 2); however, the same broad principles apply.

By graduation, you need to have become a safe and competent new (FY1) doctor. This means that you need to be very good at the skills that you will use commonly (taking a history, taking blood, cardiovascular examination, etc.) and at the skills that you may need to use less commonly but in an emergency situation (cardiopulmonary resuscitation, or taking an ECG, for example) (Figure 3.1). The next layer down covers the skills that you should be able to do under supervision (perhaps inserting a chest drain, or performing a lumbar puncture) – you should have seen and done enough of these to feel confident that you can perform these with a senior watching. Finally, there are skills that you need to know about so that you can explain them to a patient (endoscopy is just one of many examples).

Your medical school may publish lists of what skills you should gain in a number of formats: this will include being buried in course objectives ('By the end of this workshop on lung function you should be able to measure a patient's peak expiratory flow rate'), or in year objectives ('By the end of the fourth year you should be competent at conducting a female genital examination,

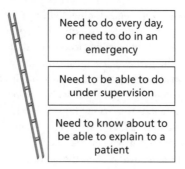

Need to do every day, or need to do in an emergency

Need to be able to do under supervision

Need to know about to be able to explain to a patient

Figure 3.1 Different levels of proficiency are required for different skills.

speculum examination, bimanual vaginal examination and perform a cervical smear') or in your overall curriculum, which may define the skills required for graduation. Many schools publish some sort of lists in the form of log-books or portfolios – for example, at Bart's and the London we published a 5-year reflective checklist of clinical and communication skills, which shows how skills build on each other year to year, we also had a year 4 logbook which included clinical skills and a statement in year 5 about skills that might be assessed in the finals.

There are some national publications too. Every few years the General Medical Council updates 'Tomorrow's doctors', which goes some way to defining minimum curriculum content (try www.gmc-uk.org, and look under 'education'). Modernising Medical Careers has published a curriculum for FY1 and FY2 (see www.mmc.nhs.uk) and other people have had a stab at it too, including the Scottish Doctor Project (www.scottishdoctor.org).

Clinical skills textbooks aren't bad either: Macleod's (Munro & Campbell, 2000) and Hutchinson's (Swash & Hutchison, 2002) are two popular ones; a look at the chapter titles gives a reasonable indication of the range of skills that you might be expected to be able to do.

So which list of skills is right? Unfortunately, you're going to have to make some judgements and build a consensus between these different sources. Forget the published lists for a moment and make your own – what skills will you need to be a newly graduated doctor? You might spend an hour or more thinking about this. Structure your list in a way that makes some sense to you (perhaps by body system, or by year of study or by level of complexity). Check some of the other lists available listed above and see what you have left out. Keep your list with you, go through it regularly, annotate it and add to it. It will become far more accurate and far more relevant than other people's lists. Perhaps your list could be the first section in your clinical skills folder.

Level of competence

We've alluded to this already: some skills you need to be pretty good at, others you should be able to do with supervision, others you need to know about. There are various different grading scales you can use between 'ignorant' and 'expert' (Table 3.1). Clearly your long-term aim is to become an expert, but at medical school you should aim to become 'good' or at least better than 'good enough' in all the core skills.

Learning clinical skills

A model for the self-directed learning of clinical skills

Learning clinical skills is very different from learning knowledge. The chances are you are pretty good at learning knowledge, with good A-levels and GSCEs. There are plenty of books on improving your study skills for knowledge, and Chapter 2 of this book adds to that large body of information. When it comes to learning clinical skills, though, there is very little out there. There are quite a few published papers talking about how the teacher should

Table 3.1 Benner's model of levels of achievement (adapted from Benner, 1984). Note that these relate to each skill, an expert at taking blood might be a novice at cardiopulmonary resuscitation

Stage 1: Novice	• Little or no prior experience of the skill
	• Tendency to focus on the skill itself rather than when to use it or what the results mean
	• Follow fixed rules that can't be adapted; this 'rule governed behaviour . . . is extremely limited and inflexible'
	• Requires full supervision and support
Stage 2: Advanced beginner	• Starts to recognise patterns from prior experience
	• Starts to use some level of judgement, able to adapt to different situations and contexts
	• Rules turn into guidelines
	• Developing dexterity
Stage 3: Competent	• Begins 'to see actions in terms of long-range goals or plans'
	• Conscious and deliberate planning
	• Able to adapt to and manage complex contexts
Stage 4: Proficient	• Understands situation as a whole, and how one skill fits into complex tasks
	• Long-term planning: how does this skill, and the way it is performed, affect the future
	• Appropriate prioritisation
	• Able to make complex judgements based on experience
Stage 5: Expert	• Accurate, intuitive, unconscious performance
	• Deep understanding of how a skill fits into the whole situation

teach clinical skills, but also plenty of papers telling us that most of the learning of skills that students do is picked up along the way, and not formally taught. How best to pick it up along the way is not mentioned.

When looking after students who struggled with clinical skills learning, it became apparent to us that there is often a problem with students not knowing *how* to learn clinical skills. Some students just read the books, without ever practising, and then seem surprised when they don't seem to be able to translate knowledge of how to perform a skill from their heads into their hands, to actually perform it. Other students practise and practise, but never get a good idea of how they should be performing a skill. Their clinical skills are often radically different from the norm, and they are unable to justify why they do each step. Finally some students mimic a video or a demonstration and practise until perfect, but without feedback they become very fluent at doing things wrong. In a recent second year Objective Structured Clinical Examination (OSCE), a number of students had practised using an online video resource for abdominal examination. They said the same words as the doctor in the video, and made the same movements, but because the camera angle hadn't been perfect, they ended up examining mostly the chest rather than the abdomen!

In response to recurrently seeing these problems, we developed a simple model for learning clinical skills (the Evans–Brown model, Fig. 3.2). It differs from all the other models in that you, the student, are central to the learning. This is how you will learn as a doctor, and this is how most of your clinical skills learning will occur as an undergraduate. The model describes three simple stages – **theory**, **practise** and **feedback**.

Building a theoretical framework on how to perform a skill
(Figure 3.2)
To perform a skill you first need to know how to perform it. To play tennis you need to know how to hold the racquet, where to stand in the court, how to strike the ball, forehand and backhand, you need to know the rules, the scoring and 101 other things, otherwise you'd just stand there, lost. Similarly for a clinical skill, you need to know how to do that skill – what steps there are to doing it. Imagine that you are going to examine a patient's abdomen – you need some knowledge of what you will be doing before you give it a go.

Often a clinician will show you their way of performing a skill, and that might act as an initial framework for you on how to do it. They are likely to tell you that their way is the best way, and it is likely that their way is the best way *for them*, but may not be the best way for you. Have a look in a clinical skills text book or two to look for other, accepted ways. Have a look perhaps on the Internet, and have a look at handouts from clinical skills sessions. They

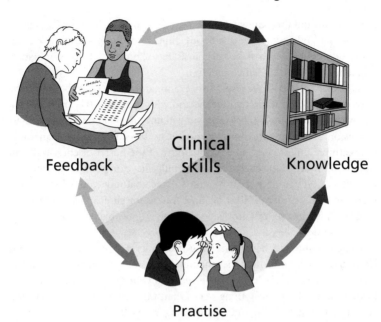

Figure 3.2 The Evans-Brown model for learning clinical skills.

are likely to be similar, but look for the similarities and particularly the differences, try and summarise the steps to perform a skill on one sheet of A4.

> *It used to really bother me that different consultants had different approaches to the same skill, and wanted me to do it their way. It took me ages to realise that over the years I would need to find the way that works for me.*
>
> Philip, fourth-year medical student

An interesting model, devised by Martina Michels (in press), identifies three different parts to the knowledge required to perform a clinical skill. The first is the **sensorimotor** aspects, the 'trick' if you like, the steps that you go through, where you put your hands, when. Most clinical skills instructions, text books and videos cover these aspects well. The second aspect is an **understanding** of the underlying principles – anatomy, physiology, even basic physics such as the principles of levers – that justifies why each step is being taken. This is where those students who just watched the video went badly wrong: they just put their hands here or there because that was what was done in the video, they didn't understand that they were supposed to be feeling for the spleen, or the liver, nor did they know where to find those organs. The final and most complex part of the knowledge is about **clinical reasoning** – making sense of your findings in order to make a diagnosis. Even knowing which examination might be appropriate in which situation.

As an example, let's take respiratory examination. You could be taught the steps of 'how to do it' pretty quickly, and with some practise and feedback you might get reasonably slick, but you will not understand testing for chest expansion unless you are aware of respiratory physiology and the anatomy of breathing; unless you know the anatomy of the posterior chest wall you will not be aware of the effect that the scapulae have on your percussion and auscultation, if you do not know your surface anatomy, you will not know if you are percussing over liver or lung. And as for clinical reasoning – you need a whole new set of knowledge to help you put together your findings into a diagnosis.

There is a difficulty here in deciding at what level to learn a skill – try and learn too much information (anatomy, physiology, pathology, clinical reasoning *as well as the* 'trick') in one go, and your brain will become overloaded and will forget everything; yet learn just the 'trick' of how to do it, and you might stop thinking and questioning yourself while you examine a patient. If you stop thinking you'll never recognise normal or abnormal.

Our recommendation is that for each skill you have three sheets of A4. The first sheet contains one side on the 'right way' (your *own* 'right way') of performing a skill (perhaps the steps for a basic knee examination) that you decide on by comparing two or three different expert sources. The second page should contain about one side of the key basic sciences that you need to support the performance of the skill (perhaps the underlying anatomy of the knee joint). The final page, which you might write only after you have started to master the skill, contains the clinical reasoning – perhaps a heading for each major condition with the key features listed, or perhaps a table of key features with their corresponding conditions. This last page is an excellent opportunity for using Cornell notes or tables (see Chapter 2).

Practice

Studies of expertise in many different disciplines suggests that about 10 000 hours of reflective, deliberate practice is required to become expert. You can't get away from this, if you want to get good, you need to practise, practise and practise some more. David Beckham has been playing football 'since he could walk'. The same goes for clinical skills, if you want to be good at taking blood, good at taking a history, good at examining a patient's respiratory system, you not only need to know how to do it, but you need to have done it again and again to transfer that knowledge from your head to your hands.

I thought that because I had taken blood pressure once, I knew how to do it. When it came to the exam I was all over the place. I think it takes quite a bit of practice to be able to do things under pressure.

Ahmed, first-year medical student

For most skills you would start by practising in **simulation**, perhaps in the skills labs, perhaps on your friends and family. An example of this is that there are two main pulses in the feet that you need to be able to feel – if you can confidently say that they are absent, then that gives a good indication that there is peripheral vascular disease, with a risk of gangrene and amputation, and you can assume that there is likely to be coronary artery disease and cerebrovascular disease too, increasing risk of a heart attack or a stroke. Feeling these pulses is difficult to begin with, but becomes easy with practice. Spend a moment to think about how many friends and family would let you examine their feet; think about how often you sit on the sofa, bored during the television adverts when you could be feeling the pulses in your feet, in your flat mates', or your loved-ones'.

Simulation has a role to play in getting you comfortable with a skill, and getting over that embarrassing clumsy stage where you're not quite sure what to do next. It is not, however, real and the only way to get good in real situations is by practising in real situations. So when you are competent enough and safe in your clinical skill, go and **practise with patients**. Examining patients is the main way that you will improve when practising your clinical skills for the rest of your life.

ASKING PATIENTS FOR CONSENT TO HELP YOU LEARN

Most medical schools now introduce students to patients at an early stage, and a substantial, perhaps majority of your time studying medicine will be on clinical attachments with patients. We write more about this clinical learning environment later in this chapter (p. 49). There is plenty written on the ethics of learning with patients, and appropriate ways of approaching it, and the BMA does a particularly nice chapter on the subject which should be available in your library, and in some institutions as an online textbook (English & Sommerville, 2004). You should have some teaching on how to approach patients and ask for their help in your learning fairly early on in your course. The key things to remember is that the patients need to know who you are, and need to willingly give informed consent to help in your learning. The information that they need to enable them to give informed consent includes what will be involved, a true estimate of how long it will take, the fact that it is only for your education and whether they say yes or no will not affect their care, and that you have the same duty of confidentiality as other professionals, namely that you will not discuss the patient outside of the clinical team or your learning group. You'll be pleased to know that most patients will be eager to help you learn. If the patient prefers that you don't examine them, thank them very politely and then move on to the next patient, they might well feel up to it next time.

> Student: *Hello, my name is John Smith, I'm a third year medical student attached to your consultant, Dr Jones. I'm currently learning how to examine the pulses in people's feet and I was wondering if I might examine your feet? It will take no more than 2 minutes and will just involve me touching your feet to try and find where the pulses are – it shouldn't be painful or anything. It's just for my learning, so no problem if you say no.*

Obviously, never pressure a patient to allow you to examine them – consent is a gift from the patient, and should be given freely, and never allow the patient to misunderstand who you are – if they say 'Yes, of course doctor', for example, correct them 'Oh no, I'm not a doctor yet, I'm a medical student, I'm *just* here to learn.' Not only is this the right and ethical thing to do, but it also stops you from getting into trouble if a patient assumes that you are qualified.

As a basic minimum you must:

- give your name (first and family name) and role;
- explain what you would like to do;
- explain that the interview is for your education only;
- explain that refusal will not affect the patient's treatment in any way;
- explain confidentiality issues e.g. where will this information go; who will see it;
- say how long it is likely to take;
- offer to come back later if the patient is tired, unwell or expecting visitors.

As a student it is never acceptable to go ahead with an interview, physical examination or procedure if the patient is uncomfortable. Equally though, medical students have a right to learn and many patients value the opportunity to talk to students and contribute to their education. Medical students are often viewed as 'neutral', that is not part of the medical establishment yet and some patients value the opportunity to talk, particularly as students may have more time than the other health professionals looking after them. Of course, this special relationship may result in a patient telling you something that they have not told the medical team and so it is essential that when talking about confidentiality you make it clear that you may share any information with the rest of the healthcare team.

Feedback

Practice on its own is, of course, not good enough. Sportsmen have coaches for good reasons: it is hard to see what you are doing while you are doing it. There are lots of ways of getting feedback: tutors are probably the most obvious candidates, an expert watching you and telling you what was good or bad. There are other ways of getting feedback too: you can ask a colleague to watch you and provide feedback, you can use video or audio taping (but beware that there are all sorts of ethical issues when using this technique with patients, so check these out first) to give yourself feedback, and you can ask the patient for feedback ('As I said earlier, I'm a medical student and just learning, can I ask how the questions I asked you about your chest pain compared with how the doctors ask about your chest pain? Did I leave anything out?' etc.).

Not only do you need to receive decent feedback, but you need to act on it too. You can find more information on giving and receiving feedback in Chapter 4. More and more medical schools are introducing portfolios and assessments that require evidence of reflection and action on feedback. You could think about adding a fourth page to each skill in your folder with two columns on – 'feedback received' and 'action taken'. Not only will this help you to ensure that you respond to feedback, but it will also give you plenty of genuine examples for your portfolio and assessments.

> I practised a lot at home on my little brother, but it was only in the retake course that I realised the importance of having other medical students giving me feedback.
>
> Katharine, third-year medical student

Learning in the clinical learning environment

Transition from secondary school to higher education is a stressful transition, requiring changes to most aspects of your life. There is plenty of research to show that transition from the classroom in higher education to the clinical learning environment (the wards, outpatients, general practice, surgical theatres) is equally, if not more, traumatic. Imagine turning up for your first full day on the wards. There is a timetable with a few sessions on – a ward round here, a clinic there. There are lots of patients. There are few or no tutors visible. There are few, if any, objectives, and little supervision. In fact, you could just go home and probably no-one would notice. This section aims to give some tips on what to do, how to make the most of what is a pretty unstructured place.

Approach to patients

We have already mentioned consent, but there are some other important issues to consider when learning with patients. Your school will discuss these with you, but as a brief introduction you should be thinking about some of the following issues. Dress is controversial but as a rule of thumb you should be dressed smartly and modestly. In practice this is likely to mean no trainers, jeans or caps, and not showing off your belly (however attractive your piercing is), your cleavage or the top of your bottom (however attractive you think your underwear is). We shouldn't need to mention that you should be clean, groomed (no stubble); you should wear deodorant but not overpowering perfume or aftershave, or too much make-up.

You should be aware of infection control, especially how to avoid spreading infections between patients – this sounds easy, but take a look on the wards and count the number of people who don't wash their hands every time, who don't have their sleeves rolled up, or who drape their tie or stethoscope over every consecutive patient – make sure that you are not one of them. Short, clean fingernails are essential for both men and women, regardless of fashion or guitar playing careers.

Respect for patients can be demonstrated in a wide range of ways. You should consider your non-verbal communication: looking uninterested, not paying attention or chewing gum will not go down well. The language that you use should reflect your developing professional practice, so think about your use of slang terms and street language. You might even ask for feedback on this from your peers and tutors.

Making the most of your tutors

We mentioned earlier on in the chapter that tutors were a good source of feedback, but the truth is that many students are observed very infrequently. Hospitals are bursting at the seams with people to teach you. The only problem is that they usually look busy, flustered and important.

One of our local professors was talking about teaching on the wards, and said: 'Those students who just sit around looking bored, I try and avoid them as much as possible, they just get in the way, but those students who are keen and enthusiastic, well, you'll do anything for them, I stay late, I miss dinner, there is nothing better than teaching someone who wants to learn – when I retire I'll really miss them.' One key skill on the wards, then, learning how to engage your tutors, how to come across as enthusiastic, interested, passionate but not pushy. This is a skill you can learn by watching others, and by a bit of trial and error, but here are some tips to start you off.

DON'T
- Sit in the corner of the ward, looking bored – it doesn't engage others.
- Just wait for teaching to happen – you need to go and find it.
- Sneak off because 'nothing's happening' – if you really, ever believe that there is nothing happening in the hospital that you can learn from, you're in the wrong career.
- Yawn and open a book half way through clinic.
- Assume that only doctors will be useful teachers – nurses are generally better at many practical skills than doctors, and have usually been taught how to teach; pharmacists are highly skilled at taking medication histories, and in spotting prescribing errors made by the doctors; the physios, the ward clerk, the list of people who you can learn from is huge.
- Assume that only the team that you are attached to are allowed to teach you. Is a psychiatrist visiting your patient? Ask if you can tag along.
- Refuse teaching because 'it's time to go home' – if someone offers to show you something interesting, go for it!

DO
- Look awake and attentive.
- Dress smartly – nothing extreme but smart and modest enough to show that you care about looking 'the part': men should avoid stubble and make sure their shirts are ironed, and women should cover their navel (even if it is bejewelled) and probably not show their underwear.
- Make the first move: 'I saw Mrs Jones when she came in through casualty, can I watch you do the lumbar puncture?' or 'I was reading about chest X-rays last night, can you tell me what you are looking at on that one?'
- Accept rejection: 'I'm far too busy to teach you right now' should get a reply 'Oh, of course, I'm sorry – is there anything I can do to help, like take forms to X-ray or something?'
- Ask for specific, achievable feedback – asking 'can you watch me while I examine Mrs Patel?' is less likely to get an enthusiastic response than 'can you watch me while I do a 5-minute cardiovascular examination on Mrs Jones, and let me know if you think I'm doing it right?'

Spot the learning opportunities

The last few paragraphs already tried to highlight that hospitals are full of learning opportunities, and that students who actively seek them out not only learn more, but also get a reputation for being keen and enthusiastic, and so get even more teaching. You can spend any dull moments trying to spot potential learning opportunities, and then go out and seize them! The list is endless. We've put a few in Table 3.2 to whet your appetite.

Table 3.2 Potential learning opportunities

Drug charts	• Go round the ward looking at everyone's drug charts, look up any drugs you don't know in the BNF
	• Ask for a blank drug chart, put a thick line through each page so it cannot be used for a real patient in error and write something like 'medical student practice' under the name. Now write up appropriate drugs for management of asthma, or angina, or heart failure, and so on. Ask one of the doctors or the ward pharmacist to comment. Tear it up or take it home when done
Drug rounds	• The nurses dispense drugs to patients several times a day – why not offer to help: you might get to learn what 'that little heart shaped pill' that patients keep talking about is, and when you sit down to learn about the drugs, you will have heard of most of them before, and even be able to pronounce them correctly
Practical skills	• Patients get their blood pressure, pulse and temperature taken between two and four times a day; on a 20-bed ward that's a lot of practice for you, and imagine how pleased the nurses or health care assistants will be for the help
Physiotherapy	• Does your patient get wheeled to physio every day? What goes on behind those big swing doors? Why not go and find out?
Radiology	• Read about interpreting radiographs; lets say chest radiographs, and then go down to the radiography department and ask what day or time they report chest radiographs; ask if you can come along and watch. The radiologists rarely have students, so you're likely to find one who is keen to teach
	• Have you ever seen a chest radiograph being taken? How about an abdominal radiograph? Or even an angiogram? What about ultrasounds? All these happen all the time in radiology departments

This list in Table 3.2 is not even a start, but will hopefully get you thinking. We've concentrated here on wards and hospitals, but you could equally write lists of opportunities for general practice, operating theatres, outpatients departments and so forth.

Summary

In this chapter we have highlighted that learning clinical skills is important, and takes deliberate, conscious effort. You will need knowledge about the skill, including how it relates to basic science and clinical reasoning, you will need to practise, practise and practise again, and that practice needs to be reflective and linked to effective feedback in order for you to learn. Clinical skills (and communication skills) are the fundamental skills of being a doctor – it is worth the investment.

References and further reading

Benner, P. (1984). *From Novice to Expert: excellence and power in clinical nursing practice.* Menlo Park, CA: Addison-Wesley.

English, V., Sommerville, A. & British Medical Association: Ethics Science & Information Division. (2004). *Medical Ethics Today: the BMA's handbook of ethics and law,* 2nd edn. London: BMJ Books.

Munro, J.F. & Campbell, I.W. (2000). *Macleod's Clinical Examination,* 10th edn. Edinburgh, Churchill Livingstone.

Swash, M. & Hutchison, R. (2002). *Hutchison's Clinical Methods,* 21st edn. Edinburgh, Saunders.

Questions and answers

Q: Tutors seem too busy to watch me perform a skill.

A: This is a common problem. You don't always need a tutor to watch you, and a colleague might be useful to watch and give you feedback. There are some things that you can do to encourage your tutors – first ensure that you have prepared your skill, so that they don't feel that they are wasting their time teaching you things you could have looked up, and second think about limiting the time that it will take. 'Can you watch me take a full history and examine this patient from head to toe – it will take about an hour' is not likely to result in success, but 'I've been practising my cranial nerve examination, I wonder if you might watch a quick 5-minute cranial nerve exam and let me know if I'm doing it right' sounds better.

Q: Every book and every tutor seems to have a different way of examining the breast – which is the right way?

A: The right way of examining a patient's breasts is a method that will be thorough, systematic, will detect pathology and will maintain the patient's dignity and comfort, and your professionalism. Check with your medical school; for exams they might expect you to perform a skill *their* way for the exams, but for real life, and practice as a doctor, try different acceptable ways of performing skills, and work out which is best for you.

Q: Not much seems to be going on, and no-one checks that I'm attending on the wards – wouldn't I be better off going home?

A: You can often get away with only turning up to the timetabled things, and slinking off home the rest of the time, but then again, if that is what you want to do, what is the point of you studying medicine?

Chapter 4 **Learning clinical communication skills**

OVERVIEW

This chapter will give you a general introduction to clinical communication skills, e.g. the communication skills you will be developing as a medical student and as a doctor. We will look at what they really are, the reasons for learning them, how to learn them at medical school and in the clinical environment.

Introduction

As a medical student (or prospective medical student) you have already shown that you are good at communicating with others by successfully passing exams, completing a UCAS application and possibly undergoing interviews for medical school or maybe a job. The good news about clinical communication skills is that they can be learned and build upon the skills you already have. They build upon the interpersonal skills, which are the general skills you use when communicating with others, such as starting and taking part in a conversation or using and reading body language, etc. Interpersonal skills are important in your communication as a medical student or doctor, and you will be building on these to develop the specialised and higher order clinical communication skills you will use as a doctor. So, don't worry too much if communication seems a challenge at the moment, with time and practice it will become clearer. Clinical communication skills will become an important part of the clinical skills toolkit you will develop over the next few years as, during your life as a doctor, you will probably conduct between 120 000 and 160 000 medical interviews with patients! (Cohen-Cole & Bird, 2000).

How to Succeed at Medical School: an essential guide to learning. By Dason Evans and Jo Brown. Published 2009 by Blackwell Publishing, ISBN: 978-1-4051-5139-9.

Why learn clinical communication skills?

Clinical communication skills are the language of medicine and the medium by which medicine is practised. They are not only essential in communicating with patients but also with colleagues, other members of the healthcare team and the wider community. At the heart of all clinical communication is the medical interview and the relationship that is built during this between doctor/student and patient. This fundamental relationship is so important and powerful that it can enhance or inhibit the patient's well-being and ability to adhere to treatment. Some would argue that this relationship is therapeutic in itself and an essential component of any treatment of a patient. Competent clinical communication skills are therefore important in providing the best possible care for patients and in enhancing your practice and satisfaction as a clinician. Sometimes students think the aim of clinical communication skills is to be 'kind' or 'nice' to patients. This is not the main aim at all, as we shall see; think rather that **effective** use of clinical communication skills will bring about an empathic, effective, efficient and satisfying interview for all concerned. But we do of course hope that kindness and politeness will always be at the centre of your professional practice as a student and as a doctor.

> *I thought communication skills classes were a waste of time as*
> *I've always been good at talking to people and had lots of*
> *experience with my previous job. I found though that they were*
> *about something different – proper professional communication.*
> *Someone told me clinical language is the equivalent of learning*
> *French!*
>
> Marcia, first-year graduate student

Clinical communication skills are evidence-based and it is through extensive research that we know that the physical and psychological health of patients are affected by clinical communication and that they play an important part in most litigation or complaints brought against doctors. They are therefore constructed from an evidence base that is as scientific as any other part of your clinical course, and in some cases is more so!

When thinking about why we learn clinical communication skills, it may be helpful to look at some important recommendations made by the General Medical Council as part of the *Tomorrow's Doctors* (GMC, 2002) document, which contains recommendations for undergraduate medical education. The GMC states that medical graduates

> *must be able to communicate clearly, sensitively and effectively with patients and*
> *their relatives and colleagues from a variety of health and social care professions*

and that

> the curriculum must stress the importance of Communication Skills and the other essential skills of medical practice.

Also, as part of the Duties of a Doctor registered with the GMC (1995), doctors must

- treat every patient politely and considerately;
- respect patients' dignity and privacy;
- listen to patients and respect their views;
- give patients information in a way they can understand;
- respect the rights of patients to be fully involved in decisions about their care.

And so the GMC supports the learning and importance of clinical communication skills and the rights of patients to be respected and treated with dignity.

At the beginning of your learning as a medical student it will be important to think about the kind of doctor you want to become and explore some of the philosophical and ethical positions around this. Developing and exploring humanistic views that value the dignity and worth of all people will provide a good foundation for building clinical communication skills. A humanist approach encourages the medical student/doctor to walk alongside the patient, acting as an expert guide but also facilitating the patient to make the best choices for themselves.

We know that during the medical interview, the patient history (the gathering of facts, information, patient ideas, concerns and expectations) that is elicited by the doctor accounts for 60–80% of the diagnosis, more than the physical examination or any investigations. So being able to conduct a competent medical interview and elicit a patient history are essential clinical skills.

Importantly for you as a medical student, Clinical Communication forms a core part of the curriculum of most medical schools in the UK and will be assessed throughout your undergraduate and postgraduate studies. They are as important as any other clinical skill and will demand your time and effort.

Assessing yourself and others

You probably know quite a lot about general communication already. As a starting point in thinking about your own skills, fill in this communication self-assessment exercise.

EXERCISE

We all need to develop self-appraisal skills if we want to have insight into our own progress and learning needs. Look at the self-appraisal questionnaire below to consider where your strengths and weaknesses lie.

Skills inventory: Think about yourself in this scheme. On a Scale from 1 (Low) to 10 (High)

How good are you at listening – really listening?

Do people generally feel comfortable with you?

How good are you at trying to put yourself in someone else's shoes?

How comfortable are you with silence?

How able are you to listen to people's feelings about their problems?

How able are you to listen to people's feelings about their distress?

How able are you to listen to people's feelings about their anger?

How good are you at explaining things to people?

How good are you at recounting events or telling stories?

Could you summarise clearly and accurately something you have just heard or read?

Are you able to tell someone honestly what you think when you know the truth may offend, upset or hurt them?

Are you able to negotiate options when there is disagreement?

(Cushing, 2003)

Now think about these three questions:
1 Consider what these answers might tell you about your strengths and weaknesses?
2 How do you know the answers you have given are correct?
3 If you dare, ask someone else that you trust to be honest to fill it out for you.
   Now you have a basis for thinking about your own communication skills and what your strengths and weaknesses are. The important thing is to work on the weaknesses as we would all rather practise the communication skills we are good at!

Another helpful exercise to spotlight effective communication skills is to:
- Think about a personal problem you have had in the past.
- Was it difficult to talk about?
- Who did you talk to about it? (friend, relative, teacher etc.)

- Why did you choose that person, what was it about them that helped you to talk?
- Can you describe the specific behaviours they used?

You may come up with a range of answers such as:
- The person was a good listener, didn't interrupt and remembered what you told them.
- You could trust this person not to gossip because you know they are discrete and never repeat private things.
- The person didn't judge you or your actions.
- The person was able to give you an honest opinion or advice.

The attitudes and skills that you identify that help you talk about your own problems usually apply to patients who want a doctor who listens well, doesn't interrupt, remembers the things they say but keeps them confidential and is honest and non-judgemental. We can transfer the communication skills that help us to our conversations with patients.

> My favourite celeb has always been Gordon Ramsay for his straight talking. When I analysed his communication style though I decided he wouldn't make a good doctor!
>
> Shaoib, first-year student

What are clinical communication skills?

Clinical communication skills cover a wide range of skills but at a basic level concern themselves with:
- eliciting a patient history
- explaining (e.g. a procedure, test or risk or giving information)
- exploring (e.g. what is going on for the patient)
- discussing informed consent
- breaking news
- negotiating (e.g. a management or treatment plan)
- passing on accurate information to colleagues (written or spoken)
- presenting a case history to colleagues.

As an illustration, let's think about a medical interview and break down the clinical communication skills under rough headings.

A check list of communication skills

Introduction and orientation	• Welcoming manner • Gives name and role • Explains purpose of the interview and any note taking • Confirms patient's comfort/agreement
Rapport	• Shows interest, respect and concern • Appropriate body language (e.g. eye contact, open posture, seating) • Matches language and energy levels
Listening skills	• Listens attentively without inappropriately interrupting • Responds to patient's answers • Picks up on patient's cues (verbal and non-verbal)
Questioning skills	• Appropriate blend of open and closed questions • Clear, jargon-free questions • Clarifies when necessary • Avoids leading questions • Keeps note taking appropriate
Empathic responses	• Reflecting back and acknowledging patients' feelings and concerns as expressed in the interview
Information giving and explaining	• Checks what patient knows/understands • Gives clear jargon-free explanations • Well paced (chunks and checks) • Invites questions, checks patient's understanding • Draws/uses diagrams where appropriate
Respecting autonomy, negotiating and shared decision-making	• Proposes options, their benefits and risks and helps the patient make their own decision • Refrains from judgment, threats or irritation
Appropriate reassurance	• Handles uncertainty appropriately • Refrains from false or premature reassurance • Offers appropriate reassurance or help
Closure	• Summarises main points to ensure everything is covered and information has been gathered accurately • If applicable, explain next step
Organisation of the interview	• Summarising • Signposting • Systematic and logical flow

(Cushing & Brown, 2001)

This checklist shows the main **process** headings of a medical interview and breaks these down into skills. The **content** of the interview is the information that is gathered or given. So we may say that some clinical communication skills are the **process** skills that enable the **content** to be gathered – essentially you can't have one without the other!

The thing to know about good clinical communication skills is that they help to build the **relationship** between the student/doctor and the patient. Without this, any medical encounter will be poor and lacking in satisfaction for both parties.

An important part of building this relationship and one of the essential principles you will learn as a medical student is the basic humanity and power of **empathy**. Empathy is the ability to walk a mile in the patient's shoes, or the appreciation, understanding and acceptance of someone else's emotional situation (Cohen-Cole & Bird, 2000), and is different from sympathy, which is about feeling sorry for someone. Empathy can be expressed in many ways and is the foundation of a patient-centred approach to care. Exploring and trying to genuinely understand what is going on in a patient's life provides a greater depth of understanding of their situation, builds a strong relationship and aids diagnosis and treatment.

How are clinical communication skills learned?

You are already reading about clinical communication skills and this is a good place to start. At the end of this chapter are some references for books that will help you look further at some of the theories and models of communication if you are interested. However, clinical communication skills cannot be learned entirely from books and must be learned by **practising or doing them**. This is sometimes called **experiential learning** and may be different from some of the learning you have done in the past. Experiential learning encourages you to actively try things out in a practical way and learn from the results. It encourages you to build upon the experience you already have and use this as a basis for developing new knowledge and skills. Think about this next activity as an example.

> **EXERCISE: AN EXAMPLE OF EXPERIENTIAL LEARNING**
>
> In order to practise your information-gathering skills, you decide to interview a friend about his recent trip to the GP surgery for a sore throat.
>
> You talk to him for about half an hour, asking questions and gathering details of his story. You might write some of this down in order to practise taking notes.

At the end of the interview, you ask your friend for some feedback about how the interview went and how he thinks you did.

He tells you that you made him feel comfortable at the start of the interview by looking interested in what he was saying. He says that you were very clear that the reason for the interview was for you to practise gathering information and that you asked clear and straightforward questions. He also tells you that he would have liked to tell you how frustrating it was to wait 45 minutes to see the GP and how apprehensive he felt when the GP took a throat swab, which actually made him want to vomit, but he didn't feel he could interrupt your flow of questions and as you were looking down to take notes he couldn't catch your eye to interrupt.

On the way home you think about and reflect on the interview. You realise that you were successful in gathering information from your friend but that you got so carried away with asking him your questions and taking notes that you didn't give him an opportunity to tell you about the things that were important for him. You decide that next time you interview someone, you will start by asking them to tell their story first, before asking your questions and so start with what is most important for them.

You also decide to spend less time looking down at your notes and more time maintaining eye contact to pick up body language clues.

Using role play to learn clinical communication skills

Many medical schools use role play as part of experiential learning. Role play allows you to try out or practise a patient interview in a simulated setting (a classroom or group learning room) with a simulated patient (an actor, another student or sometimes a specially trained patient). A role play group should be thought of as a safe laboratory for experimenting where any explosions will be harmless! And so don't be afraid to try things out, experiment and see what works best for you as this is a golden opportunity and there is no such thing as a perfect role play. We all have different ways of learning and some people may feel less comfortable about learning with role play, but just resolve to give it a go, jump in at the deep end and see how it feels. Many people who feel apprehensive at the start go on to really enjoy and value role play as an effective way of learning clinical communication skills. In fact, all the research tells us that experiential learning and role play are the best ways to learn clinical communication skills and that it is important to practise these skills as much as possible. As we've already mentioned, it takes 10,000 hours of deliberate, reflective practice to become an expert and at least 100 hours until you become reasonably competent at a skill (Anderson, 1982;

Bruning *et al.*, 2004). Clinical communication skills are no different and so practise, practise, practise makes perfect!

The usual set-up is for a role play session to be carried out in a small group with a tutor. There is usually a predetermined patient scenario that has been written to allow particular skills in a relevant clinical situation to be practised. In its simplest form, each student tries out a role with an actor or simulated patient for a short time and then gets feedback on their performance from others in the group. Sometimes there is an opportunity to re-do parts of a role play to see if things turn out differently and sometimes the role play can be recorded on video or DVD to allow the role player to see themselves in a particular situation. Seeing yourself on video can be a nerve-wracking experience the first time, but students rate this highly as a very useful learning experience. You often have to play the video/DVD several times until you get over seeing and hearing yourself on screen and can look at what is actually happening in the role play.

Feedback

Feedback is an essential part of role play; in fact, you cannot have one without the other. We all need feedback from others to get a different perspective on our performance and just as we saw in the experiential learning example, often we are not aware of some of our own behaviours and how others may see or be affected by these. Giving and receiving feedback should be an honest and constructive experience. Feedback is not about character assassination or comments of a personal nature, but should be focused on a person's **behaviour** in a given situation, helping them to develop new perspectives or behaviours if appropriate.

An example of this may be that you have watched a fellow student talking to a patient and noticed that the patient was finding it difficult to hear because the student was speaking so softly. The feedback you may want to give would be centred on the student speaking louder and also watching the patient to pick up cues that they found it difficult to hear; this feedback would allow the student to think about their behaviour next time and possibly change it. What you would *not* give feedback on is the student's voice itself, which is personal, probably can't be changed and will result in them feeling hurt or personally criticised.

Behaviours and skills are not in themselves 'good' or 'bad' – it depends on the effect they have and if they are achieving the objectives. When giving someone feedback, remind yourself to look at what worked well at the same time as what might be improved, and consider suggestions for how to improve things. This is important for a reason other than kindness, as at any given moment we can only put a certain amount of energy toward changing ourselves. It is a help to know what we already do that works well and therefore doesn't need to be looked at. We can then concentrate more easily on other suggestions for change.

SOME FEEDBACK TIPS

- Do whenever possible allow the person whose skills are being evaluated to do a self-critique first. Usually, people in this position are very critical, and find it difficult to describe what they have done well. Although they may need to deal with any problem they experienced, it is also important to point out aspects that worked well.

- When you give feedback, you may find that all you have to do is emphasise points already made by the person whose skills are being discussed. If not, make two or three comments, but always by describing (behaviourally) what you saw, why you think it is not the best way (refer to the effect it had on the patient) and what you suggest would be an improvement. Try to make it a habit to write down some of your comments so that the person can read them later.

- Do always focus on what you see by describing behaviours. For example, rather than saying something general like 'You're doing OK', try something specific like 'I liked the way you checked to make sure Mrs Jones understood your explanation'.

- There is a difference between the intention behind our behaviours and the effect they have. For example rather than say 'You made that patient embarrassed' (which may not have been the intention), try something like 'When you . . . , I thought the patient looked embarrassed'.

- Remember that **all feedback is subjective** and the person receiving it may disagree.

(Cushing, 2000)

So, it is important to be specific when giving feedback, concentrate on a particular part of an interview and perhaps write down some of the words that are said – this will aid your memory. It is also important not to overwhelm people with lots of feedback that they probably won't remember! Try to limit feedback to the three most important things you saw.

When I saw myself on DVD doing a role play I couldn't believe how awful I looked and sounded – I had to go over it with friends lots of times. Eventually I could see what I was doing and it was really helpful to have that perspective.

Phoebe, third-year student

Feedback can be a tricky skill to get right and needs practise: we all enjoy giving positive feedback but find negative feedback more difficult. Interestingly, students say they value honest feedback from colleagues and teachers above all else and find it the most helpful way to learn. Working in small groups with colleagues allows you to develop an honest and trusting group relationship that fosters constructive and honest feedback.

Giving and receiving feedback will be important skills to develop over your medical training as they will not just be needed for role play but for a range of things throughout the rest of your professional life. Someone who regularly gives and receives feedback will be in tune with others and not just relying on their own thoughts and opinions.

Learning clinical communication skills in the clinical environment

At some point in your course you will begin to learn and take part in the clinical environments of hospital wards, outpatient clinics and general practice and primary care. For some people this will be the most exciting and rewarding part of their course and for others it may seem quite unstructured and therefore a little daunting. The work you may have done experientially will be a good preparation and foundation for this part of the course where you will be talking to and learning from real patients.

The clinical environment offers wonderful learning opportunities, but sometimes it is difficult to recognise them, particularly if you are the kind of person who likes very structured activities with a tutor taking the lead. We remember our own experiences of going on to a ward for the first time and not knowing where to physically 'be' for most of the time. Everyone seemed to be very busy, very confident and knew what they were doing: it took a few weeks to settle in and find our places in this new world. Everyone feels like this! The vital thing is to realise that you have to make learning opportunities for yourself as clinicians will have competing priorities and won't be able to offer support all the time. It may be helpful to plan your day around the structures that already exist, such as ward rounds, surgeries and clinics.

Ask yourself:

- How can I prepare for the upcoming ward round/surgery/clinic?
- Which patients should I be talking to and examining today?
- How will I get feedback on what I am doing today?
- How will I record what I have learned today?
- Which other members of the healthcare team should I be working with today?

At this point it is important to mention informed consent and patient rights. You will remember that these were more fully written about in the clinical skills section.

In the clinical environment you will be introduced to 'clerking', which is taking a full history and performing a full examination of a patient. At first this will take quite a while and you will need lots of practise. Aim to fully clerk five patients per week and this will soon add up to a substantial number – remember each skill takes 100 hours of practice in order to achieve a minimal competency. By interviewing patients regularly you will learn how to approach them and build rapport, how to find out about their story and record this accurately, how to elicit their concerns and fears and find out about their health beliefs and how to examine them competently.

The more you talk to patients and immerse yourself in the clinical environment the easier things will become. If you are the kind of person who finds it difficult to approach a patient or strike up a conversation, try to prepare for this in advance by **visualising** what you will do.

- Visualise yourself walking over to the patient.
- Visualise how you will greet them – what words will you use?
- How will you go through the steps of consent – what words will you use?
- Will you ask for permission to sit down?
- What opening line will you start off with – the weather, their journey, photos on the locker, asking about lunch?

This technique is useful for preparing yourself. It may also be helpful to jot down the areas you would like to talk to them about on your pad to act as an *aide-memoire*. A simple history template is sometimes helpful:

- the presenting problem(s)
- history of the presenting problem(s)
- past medical history
- family history
- medication history
- social history.
- review of systems

A tip here is not to prepare the questions you are going to ask but simply to be curious about your patient and their story and really listen to what they tell you. Often students stop listening and miss information because they are concentrating on the next question they are going to ask. Listening is one of the most important clinical communication skills. You also should avoid asking 'checklist' questions guided by the history template – patients' do not tell their story according to a checklist. Your job is to **map their story** onto a clinical template rather than the other way round.

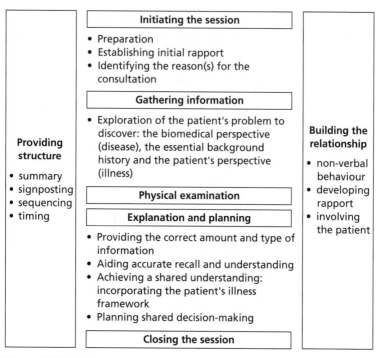

Figure 4.1 *The Calgary Cambridge Guide*: A Guide to the Medical Interview.

This is a good point to introduce you to two models for taking a patient history. Model 1 (Figure 4.1) is a simplified version of the *Calgary Cambridge Guide* (Kurtz *et al.*, 1998), which breaks the medical interview down into the five steps: initiating the session, gathering information, the physical examination, explanation and planning, and closing the session. At the same time it provides two pillars that run through the five steps and outline the skills that provide structure for the interview and build the relationship with the patient. You may want to use this as a template for your interviews with patients.

Model 2 (Figure 4.2; McWhinney, 1989) is the patient-centred clinical interview, which presents the 'doctor's agenda' and the 'patient's agenda' as two parallel frameworks that aim to be integrated at the end of the medical interview. Again, the communication or **process** skills are made clear. These two models will provide you with a firm foundation for taking a patient history and you may like to experiment using both to see how they fit with your particular interviewing style.

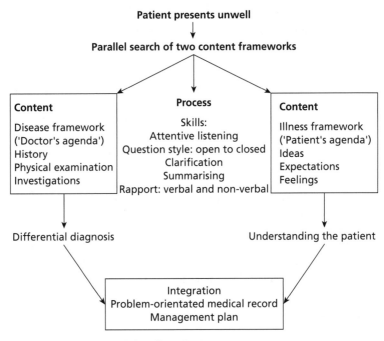

Figure 4.2 Patient-centred clinical interview.

Where possible and appropriate, try to interview patients in pairs initially. This allows one of you to talk to the patient while the other observes and gives feedback. If you are feeling really brave you could also ask the patient to give you some feedback. Remember that feedback is the key to good clinical communication skills and that the more you receive, the better and more skilled you become. Try to get feedback from a variety of people so that you get a wide perspective on your skills. It will be important to ask the senior doctors and nurses to watch you for a few minutes with a patient and then give you feedback. You may like to ask them for specific feedback; for example, supposing you have identified that you have a tendency to inappropriately interrupt patients before they have finished telling you something, or that you find it difficult to use open questions when taking a patient history, ask for specific feedback about these, it can be really helpful to pinpoint specific things. But you must also bear in mind that *all* feedback is subjective and opinion-based, which is why gathering a variety of views helps to maintain a balance.

> *One of my interviews in the third year was with a patient who cried when we talked about his wife who had recently died. I felt useless at the time,*

but the next day when I went back he said he was comforted by me just listening to him and thought I would make a good doctor

Muna, fourth-year student

Not all interviews with patients need be long or very formal. In some settings such as outpatient clinics or GP surgeries it may only be possible to speak to patients for a short time. Gathering and grabbing all opportunities to talk to patients is the vital thing and will help you build up an extensive and varied experience base. A useful tip is to keep a patient interview diary (ensuring you do not use patient names or identifiers), where you write down the various interviews you conduct, what were the strengths and weaknesses and what you have learned from these and what to try out next. It may also be helpful to record the particular types of histories or examinations you have done to make sure you have a wide experience, for example if you have spent some time interviewing patients about their asthma, perhaps you should aim to do the same with patients who have diabetes or are about to undergo a procedure or operation of some kind. This way you have a clinical log as well as a reflective journal of clinical communication skills.

Summary

In this section we have looked at the definition of clinical communication skills, why they are used and how they can be developed and practised in a simulated setting. We have looked at ways of applying them in a clinical environment with real patients and at the importance of feedback to their development. We have looked also at the doctor/student–patient relationship and the importance of empathy to this.

- Clinical communication skills are not about being 'kind' or 'nice' to patients.
- Good clinical communication is essential to clinical competence.
- Clinical communication skills are evidence based.
- Listening and curiosity are key communication skills.
- Practice and feedback are essential to the development of competent clinical communication skills.

References and further reading

Anderson, J.R. (1982). Acquistion of cognitive skill. *Psychological Review* 89: 369–406.

Bruning, R.H., Schraw, G.J., Norby, M.M. & Ronning, R.R. (2004). *Cognitive Psychology and Instruction*, 4 edn. Upper Saddle River, N.J., Pearson/Merrill/Prentice Hall.

Cohen-Cole, S.A. & Bird, J. (2000). *The Medical Interview: the three-function approach*, 2nd edn. St. Louis, MO, Mosby.

Cushing, A.M. (2000). *Guidelines on Giving Feedback*. London, Barts and the London School of Medicine and Dentistry.

Cushing, A.M. (2003). *A Communication Skills Self-Assessment Form*. London, Barts and the London School of Medicine and Dentistry.

Cushing, A.M, & Brown, J. (2001). *Communication Skills Feedback Form*. London, Barts and the London School of Medicine and Dentistry, p. 1.

General Medical Council. (1995). *Duties of a Doctor: guidance from the General Medical Council*. London, General Medical Council.

General Medical Council. (2002). *Tomorrow's Doctors: recommendations on undergraduate medical education*. London, General Medical Council.

Kurtz, S.M., Silverman, J.D. & Draper, J. (1998). *Teaching and Learning Communication skills in Medicine*. Abingdon, Radcliffe Medical.

McWhinney, I. (1989). *The Need for Transformed Clinical Method in Communicating with Medical Patients*. Newbury Park, CA: Sage Publications.

Silverman, J.D., Kurtz, S.M., Draper, J., Kurtz, S.M.T. (2005). Learning Communication Skills in Medicine, 2nd edn. *Skills for Communicating with Patients*, Oxford, Radcliffe Pub.

Questions and answers

Q: I find it difficult to disturb patients to talk to them as I cannot help with their treatment.

A: It is quite true that talking to patients is for the purpose of helping your learning and education, but patients quite often enjoy talking to students and may feel this is a way of practically helping with your education. It is also true that you have a right to be a learner and that although the needs of the patient must be uppermost, the best way for you to learn is by talking and practising.

Q: I find the wards quite bewildering. I never know which patients to talk to, or whether it is OK for me to talk to them?

Everyone feels like this at the beginning. The important thing is to agree with your clinical supervisor which patients you will approach as he/she will be able to guide you and may want you to look at specific patients, perhaps because there is a ward round coming up or because the patient is about to return home, etc. The vital thing is to treat the clinical environment as a place of learning and try to gain as much experience as possible.

Q: A patient that I particularly got on with told me something she had not told the doctor.

A: This sometimes happens which is why it is important that when you obtain consent to interview a patient that you explain you cannot guarantee confidentiality between you, but that any information will be shared within the healthcare team. Importantly though it will *not* be shared *outside* the healthcare team, which includes the patients family, friends or work etc. You will need to discuss any additional information you gather about a patient with their supervising clinician.

Q: *It takes me a long time to take a patient history, sometimes over an hour. Nobody else seems to take this long.*

A: At the beginning it is common to take a long time to interview a patient. Over time, you will become more comfortable with the process and more proficient at interviewing or examining a patient. Enjoy this time and make the most of being with patients in an unpressured time frame.

Q: *Sometimes it feels like I am prying into the patient's private life when I take a history.*

A: This is a common and understandable concern but there is a clinical *reason* for asking a patient personal questions. In the normal run of things a patient would not dream of sharing such information with you, but as a medical student you are in a privileged position in which you are able to ask patients in-depth questions about their lives. You seek out this information in order to take a full and competent clinical history, it is not done as part of curiosity or prying but as a clinical skill.

Chapter 5 **Working in a group**

OVERVIEW

This chapter gives you some useful tips on how to build and maintain productive group work. Group work is important in medicine both as an undergraduate and as a doctor, so we hope that this chapter will help act as a springboard for effective team working and team learning for many years to come.

Introduction

As a medical student and as a doctor, for the rest of your professional life, you will be required to study and work with others. We have already highlighted (Chapter 4) the importance of working in a study group, but we haven't given you much guidance on how to get one together, how to make it work. This chapter will help you identify your personal preferences when it comes to group work and will describe some of the pros and cons. We will dip into some practical theory from educational psychology to consider why and how things can go wrong, and what the key strategies are for making it go right.

The second half of this chapter will look at the specific challenges of problem-based learning groups, self-study groups and interprofessional learning. You will also find useful advice relevant to study groups for clinical skills in Chapter 3 and clinical communication skills in Chapter 4.

What do you think?

Different people have very different perspectives on learning in a group. Some love it, some hate it. This perspective is partly due to some level of inbuilt preference (whether from nature or nurture, some people tend to be 'loners'), but is largely due to past experience. Consider the exercise you did

How to Succeed at Medical School: an essential guide to learning. By Dason Evans and Jo Brown. Published 2009 by Blackwell Publishing, ISBN: 978-1-4051-5139-9.

in Chapter 1, p. 7. How did you answer the question on group work? Think back to a typical example of group work from your past, try to recall the session in your mind, or even in writing. Ask yourself the following questions:

- What was the task?
  - In what way did the nature of the task affect how the group worked together?
- What about the make-up of the group?
- What were the behaviours between people in the group?
  - Which were helpful?
  - Which were unhelpful?
  - Were any behaviours particularly destructive?
  - What did the group do about these?

Spend another couple of minutes thinking about the following question:

- What would be the characteristics of a task that encouraged productive group-work?
- What would be the perfect list of different characters or personalities or skills in the group for productive collaboration? You might want, for example, someone who is good at finding information, someone else who is good at motivating the group. What others can you think of?

Your prior experience is important; if you have had positive experiences in the past then you are likely to be the sort of person who will engage positively with future experiences. The opposite is true too. This is important to be aware of – other members of the group might behave in ways that help or hinder the group's productivity, but so do you. Go back to the questions above, and consider what behaviours that you had in the group, and what effect it had.

> *Some friends invited me to join their study group for clinical skills.*
> *We set a topic in advance, but I didn't really prepare. They ended up*
> *teaching me and one of them got quite angry that they were only*
> *covering the basics, and I got angry back. I never went back, which is a*
> *shame – its hard to learn clinical skills on your own.*
>
> Colum, first-year medical student

Pros and cons

There are, of course, pros and cons to working in a group. Some are real; others are more subjective. Some are fixed whereas others can be influenced in ways that we will discuss below. We don't plan to produce an exhaustive list here, and we're sure that you could add more, but we will try and provide a balanced list (Tables 5.1 and 5.2).

Table 5.1 Advantages of working in a group

Collective knowledge is more than individual knowledge	You will never know everything, others will always know things that you don't know, and you will always know things that others don't know. You can always learn from others
Collective skills are more than individual skills	As you will see later, different people tend to have different roles within a group. You may not be as good at finding information as one of your peers, but perhaps you are better at spotting links across topics or getting an overview or 'helicopter view' of the topic. Together you are stronger than apart
Learning through teaching	One of the best ways of checking that you understand something is by explaining it to someone else; if you can do this, and answer their questions, it will consolidate the facts in your head much more deeply
Depth and breadth	We have mentioned the problem of depth and breadth quite a lot. Throughout your time at medical school you will struggle with knowing when you know enough. The three main ways of telling are through exam results (too late), by looking at the learning objectives (often not specific enough) and by measuring yourself against your peers
Hidden curriculum	For good or for bad, the grapevine carries a lot of information about the curriculum. Students who work alone are often unaware of things that everyone else knows. ('I just didn't know what to expect for the exam' when every other student in the school knew what the questions were last year and the year before)
Motivation and empathy	We all have bad days. Days that we don't seem to be able to get round to doing work, that nothing seems to make sense. If someone you trust tells you that they had a similar experience last week, then you might decide to give it another go tomorrow. Perhaps they also struggled with the same topic, and found a really useful way of looking at it that will help you too
Divide and conquer	For some tasks (not all tasks), many hands really can make light work, especially if you coordinate your efforts well. Often tasks can be divided up between you, and then recombined to make a good finished product far more quickly and easily than it would take one person alone

Table 5.2 Disadvantages of working in a group

You know a lot more than them	When you know a lot more than the rest of the group on a topic, then you can spend a disproportionate amount of time explaining very basic things when you could be using that time more productively alone
You know a lot less than the rest	If most people in the group seem to know a lot more about the topic than you, the level of discussion can be so high that you have trouble following. You might just sit there, listening to a foreign language, and get frustrated at the waste of time, or demoralised at your lack of knowledge
Disorder and disharmony	We have all worked in groups where people tended to shout each other down a lot, play one-upmanship and try and win points over the others. Often this is a normal stage that a group can go through (see Table 5.4), but sometimes the group can be stuck in chaos and struggle to be productive
Individual behaviours	Sometimes one or two individuals can have behaviours that make it difficult for the group to function. Perhaps they get angry, or put others down. They often don't realise, but sometimes they do
Not sharing the workload	Colum's quote highlights a relatively common phenomenon when some members of a group don't 'carry their weight'. If they never or rarely prepare, they become seen as 'hangers on', and resentment can start to build in the group

Of course, working in a group is not all roses, and you have probably come across some difficulties and disadvantages; we list some typical problematic situations in Table 5.2.

The difficult truth

Love them or hate them, the clean and simple truth is that you will need to learn to work in a group. At medical school you will benefit from doing some of your study in a group (you can't learn clinical or communication skills without it, for example), and for the rest of your professional life you will be working in teams.

The people in these teams will not always be people who you would choose for friends, but you will need to learn to value them for their strengths and recognise and support their areas of weakness, and they should do the same for you. Similarly, in study groups, you may not always work with people who are your friends, but you can still be amazingly productive.

We hope that we have convinced you that you will need to work in groups, that there are advantages and that it isn't always plain sailing. The rest of this chapter looks at how you might help the group to be as productive as possible.

Roles within a group

Back in the 1980's, Dr Raymond Meredith Belbin published his investigation of management teams in industry. His work identified that for a team to work productively people took on different roles within the team, with some people taking on more than one role. He came up with some rather strange names for the different roles, which we will try and summarise here (Table 5.3). As you read through them, see if you can identify with them from teams that you have worked or studied in.

Table 5.3 Belbin's model of team roles

Chairman/coordinator	This role involves coordinating the others, delegating the right jobs to the right people, providing focus on the task
Shaper/motivator	Shapers tend to be full of enthusiasm and motivation for the task. They are keen to 'win' and their passion overflows to others, they can be quite aggressive in their aim to achieve
Plant	These are bright, intellectual lateral thinkers. They are great at coming up with ideas, different ways of doing things
Monitor/evaluator	People in this role are those who keep an eye on deadlines, and progression towards them. They will think things through and propose the most sensible path. Often they are pragmatic, and may be a little cynical
Company worker	This is the role that gets the work done; they are loyal to the team and get the work done on time
Team worker	This role is interested in building the team spirit and keeping everything running smoothly. They are the diplomats and tend not to take sides
Completer/finisher	This role is interesting. It involves producing a suitable finished product – dotting the i's and crossing the t's, checking the spelling. Ironically, their high standards can frustrate others and actually lead to delays in completion (so not, perhaps, the best name)
Resource investigator	This role involves actively seeking out sources of information, external contacts, and building networks outside of the team

Adapted from Watkins & Gibson-Sweet (1997).

The interesting thing about Belbin's model is that not only can one person play more than one role within a team, but that they may play different roles in different teams. Also, people tend to have roles that they are good at, and roles that they find more difficult. Imagine that you are a perfectionist who prefers to do things right. You will probably be comfortable putting things together into a final product (completer–finisher) and might be quite reasonable at many of the other roles too, but you will find it more difficult to delegate, and so might find it harder work to fill a coordinator role.

This Belbin model is not perfect, and our brief description of it is rather superficial, but it does give a framework with which to look at a group that you are working in, and consider some of the reasons that there might be challenges.

Imagine the following scenario: four of you have been selected to produce a poster on health in the local community.

- If none of you take on the role of resource investigator, then how will you find the data that you need?
- If no-one takes on a coordinator role, then how will you avoid everyone doing the same things?
- If everyone takes on a coordinator role, how will you ever agree on what needs to be done?
- If no-one in the group has attention to keeping the team together, then who will ease things over when you can't agree on a background colour for the poster?

The Belbin roles allow you to do more than just understand why things are going wrong. You can actively use this framework to ensure that the group becomes productive

- You might consciously decide to invite people to join the group who you think will fill in the gaps – if you don't have an obsessive–compulsive proofreading completer–finisher in the group, and your posters tend to look rather tatty, perhaps you could invite one to join you, regardless of whether you like their company or not.
- You might use the Belbin framework to have a discussion in your group – perhaps you are all keen to lead, and none to follow, if you can talk about this, perhaps you could rotate the role of coordinator.
- You might also use the framework to personally think how you will work within the group. You are likely to be pretty good at four or more of the roles, and probably reasonably good at another two or so. Imagine that no-one in your group is very good at keeping the team spirit up, and you know that with some effort you can do that, you might decide to throw yourself into that role, even though it isn't your strongest preference.

Watkins and Gibson-Sweet's article (1997) is a good starting point if you wish to read more. They even give a different analogy of teamwork, useful for those who find Belbin's roles too abstract.

Group dynamic, group development

Groups don't start functioning at 100% capacity straight away. They often go through a rocky period in the first few meetings. You know this from experience, and Bruce Tuckman formally described it in 1965. He described four stages that a group goes through before they start 'performing' (Table 5.4).

The strange thing about the model in Table 5.4 is that it appears to be true. Almost all groups seem to go through these stages, although some get stuck at one stage or another.

The relevance to you is twofold. First, if on the second or third time your group meets, people seem to stop getting on, perhaps they start talking each other down and argue a bit, then you can be reassured that this tends to happen, and most groups will move on to start performing within a couple more meetings. In addition, though, you might think about how you might help a 'storming' group to move on to a more productive stage. Your group tutor (if you have one) should also help, but your role within the group will put you in a position of influence. Consider what you have read about feedback (Chapter 4) and reflection (Chapter 7), and use this to provide feedback for

Table 5.4 Bruce Tuckman's four stages of team development

Forming	At this stage, members of the group are polite and try to understand each other and the unwritten rules within the group. They avoid conflict and their comments tend to be generic or ambiguous so as not to risk disagreement
Storming	The politeness ends here, and the conflict begins. This might be conflict about the right way of pursuing the task, or vying for leadership or respect within the group. Members are more willing to disagree, and conflict may range from members talking each other down all the way to displays of anger
Norming	In this stage the group has learnt the unspoken rules of how they will work together, they develop trust and respect and become a true team
Performing	Having successfully navigated the previous three stages, the group become truly productive

Adapted from Westberg & Jason (1996).

the group, and stimulate them to think about the processes going on. Examples might include:

- *'I notice that we tend to keep interrupting each other a lot, and we seem to lose out on a lot of information by not listening, could we think about some ground rules for the group?'*
- *'We seemed to be getting along so well last week, I wonder what was different between then and now.'*

Other factors affecting learning in a group

There is a lot of evidence from educational psychology that various factors other than development of group dynamic and roles within a group also influence the productivity of the group. In this section we will list them, give brief descriptions and some practical suggestions.

Products/goals

Goals that are more concrete tend to produce more interaction (although unfortunately also less breadth of learning), so you might wish to help your group make its goals as concrete as possible.

- 'So to summarise, when we meet next Thursday we will all be able list all the causes of clubbing and we will construct a table of what other clinical features would point us to each of those diagnoses.'

  Goals that are shared between members of the group tend to be better than goals that are divided up between individuals. Although the goals should be shared, individuals should still be accountable within the group.

- You might start a session going round members of the group to find out how they prepared for the session. Often this is in the form of people talking about what sources of information they found.

  The nature of the task itself seems important, with tasks that require everyone's input having a better effect on group interaction. Concept maps, for example, seem to be better than a poster or an essay that one person could make on their own.

- Work hard to ensure that everyone has input to the final product.

Individual factors and positive interdependence

Although prior knowledge is important, for a group to learn and grow effectively together they should have a similar level of prior knowledge. We hinted at this when talking about the cons of group work. Although the members of the group don't need the same prior knowledge, clearly if one person is an expert and the others are novices the session will become simply a teaching session, at the cost of group motivation and the importance of debate, discussion and elaboration.

- Try to ensure a similar level of prior knowledge – encourage members to do the study that they agreed before the session, and discourage those who try to read ahead of everyone else.

     Positive interdependence is a term used to mean that everyone in the group should require the others to complete the task, or to complete the task well. Groups that appreciate that their results are better because of the different members of the group tend to continue to perform well.
- Try and ensure that the goals are owned by everyone (as above).
- Help the group to consider the strengths of its members – perhaps you could say something positive about everyone's contribution.

Behaviour within the group

If you read Chapter 2 you will not be surprised that **asking questions** (especially questions that encourage deep understanding), elaboration and trying to build links with other learning will result in deeper learning and better group performance.

Ask questions, be curious, try and apply the knowledge that you are sharing and try and link with other learning. Ensure that you are all actively learning in the group.

> *Someone in my group kept asking 'why' and we really found it
> irritating to begin with, she persevered and suddenly we realised that
> we couldn't really explain the things we were saying, we didn't
> understand as deeply as we had thought. We were quite shocked and
> had to go back to the books. I now think that 'why' is one of the most
> powerful questions.*
>
> > Jason, third-year graduate entrants' programme student

Whereas emotional conflict can be quite destructive in a group, **cognitive conflict** can help ensure deep learning and a common understanding. Cognitive conflict refers to a disagreement on a thinking, rather than an emotional, level, and it tends to stimulate motivation, curiosity and reflection.

- Ask questions that will stimulate curiosity and challenge fixed views, such as: 'If, as we read, a fasting blood glucose of ≥ 7.0 mmol/L diagnoses diabetes, but why 7.0 rather than 6.9 or 7.2?'

> *'I love a good debate, and so did the others in my group, we learnt a lot by
> disagreeing with each other.'*
>
> > Abdul, final-year medical student

Interestingly, the more that the interaction in the group is **structured**, the better the learning outcomes tend to be (but at the cost of free thought). This might well be part of the advantages of some of the highly structured models of collaborative learning such as problem-based learning, but it can also work to your advantage in less formal settings.

- Consider setting some ground rules for how the group wants to work. Perhaps for revision sessions you will agree to always start with a brainstorming session on the topic, followed by a review of the learning objectives set by the school, and you follow that up with making up some questions individually and trying to write model answers for them as a group. You will find these sessions much more productive than just turning up to 'revise diabetes'.

Understanding **other people's point of view** is one of the most important parts of working in a group. We talked about empathy with patients in the chapter on clinical communication, and empathy with others in your study group is just as important. Often emotional conflicts occur because individuals are more interested in pushing their own point of view rather than truly trying to build a consensus. For a consensus to form, everyone needs to see each other's perspective and try and see how it relates to each of the other members' perspective.

- If you find that the conversation keeps jumping – student A makes point X, student B makes point Y, which is unrelated to point X and student C interrupts to make a different point – then try proposing this simple exercise: whenever anyone speaks, they summarise what the last person said, and build on it. Give it a try, it is harder than it sounds!
- If different opinions are flying wildly around the group, consider stepping out of your own opinions, and into a facilitative role. For example:
  'This is interesting, we seem to have three different opinions here. If I can just summarise where I think we are at, Jacob seems to argue heavily that prostitution' should be legalised so that it can be regulated, but Malini thinks that this will just encourage an explosion in an already crime-ridden area. It seems to me that there was also a second debate, more focused on the women themselves, with Peter keen that they become destigmatised and supported, and I think the only way that he saw this happening was through legalisation. Could we agree that that summary is broadly what we have covered so far? OK, so should we brainstorm what we know about regulation, association with crime and stigmatisation in prostitution?

You won't be surprised to hear that just with individual learning, group learning is driven by **motivation**. Some are motivated externally (we have to work together to get this assignment done) whereas others are driven by interest in the topic, or the feeling of unity with the group, or by the interactions and cognitive conflicts within the group (Abdul's quote above, for example). If you can maximise this motivation, in yourself and others, the group is more likely to be productive.

• Consider talking about what motivates you and starting a discussion. If everyone knows that you are interested especially in the pure science, and another group member is more motivated by relevance to patient care, then you can make sure that your discussions are tailored for both of you.

Special cases

Problem-Based Learning

Problem-based learning (PBL) is simply a structured way of going about group work. There is some evidence that students who learn in this way are more highly motivated, learn more deeply and integrate their knowledge together more effectively. Because of this, there are plenty of medical schools where the vast majority of the information that students learn is learnt through PBL, your school might be one of them. Medical Educationalists are passionate about PBL (they either love it or hate it) and, it probably goes without saying, there are lots of different flavours of PBL, with their different proponents arguing that theirs is 'the' right way. Some schools use the term case-based learning (CBL) to refer to the sort of learning that we are talking about here, but others use case-based learning to mean something rather different.

The PBL group is made up of students (including a chairperson and a scribe) and a tutor. There are perhaps six to eight students in a group, sometimes more, and one takes the role of chairperson. This 'chair' keeps order, guides the group through the steps of PBL and ensures that everyone has their say. A different student takes the role of scribe – writing things up on a board, usually a whiteboard, and capturing the discussion. The scribe has quite a position of power, and of responsibility, as they can direct how things go by the way that they write things down. Innovative scribes, who use colours, concept maps, flow diagrams, tend to drive innovation in the group. Scribes who just tend to write lists can sometimes have a very negative effect on the group. The most remarkable thing about PBL is the role of the tutor. The tutor does not teach. He or she should act as a facilitator only, keeping in the background, supporting the chair and scribe, occasionally asking a question or nudging the topic gently one way or another, and sometimes challenging unhelpful group behaviours.

The learning in the group centres on a problem, and a structured way of thinking about that problem. The problem itself is usually something relevant to the topic, and often relates to a realistic context. Good problems should stimulate curiosity and motivation, and make the students puzzled, keen to find a solution. Good problems should be difficult or even impossible to 'solve' – the learning comes in thinking and debating and reading and testing hypotheses, not in finding the 'right' answer.

We stated that there were different flavours of PBL, here we will run through the seven-jump process that is used in many medical schools in the UK. It came to the UK from Canada via Maastricht in the Netherlands, and there is a huge amount of educational research about it. If you are interested, try putting 'problem-based learning' into a PubMed search.

Step (jump) 1: Clarifying terms

This is an interesting step. The group reads through the problem statement, which is often a paragraph or more, and identify any words or phrases that anyone in the group doesn't understand fully. Either other members of the group can help provide a definition, or the group can list the word or statement as something that they will need to look up. Clearly, this is an important step because the group needs to have the same understanding of the words in the problem to be able to discuss it, but in addition, in some research at Barts and the London and Kings, we have found that this stage seems to help allow students to feel safe to admit 'not knowing' right at the beginning of the session. This was valued, and felt to be different from a tutor-led tutorial.

Step 2: Define the issues

In this step, the students try and list as many issues as they can see in the problem – perhaps 'What is diabetes? Why was this patient started on insulin? What would have happened if she hadn't had treatment? Why didn't she take her insulin as prescribed?' etc. There are often main issues and sub-issues, sometimes there are a number of different angles (perhaps a biomedical, a sociological, a legal perspective).

Note that many texts use the word 'problems' rather than 'issues' for this step, but we have noticed that this can cause confusion between the initial problem ('problem statement'), and then breaking that down into further 'problems', if you see what we mean. We will stick with 'issues' for clarity.

Step 3: Brainstorm/analyse the issues

Here the group takes each issue in turn and brainstorms freely on what they know about it. Personal experience, prior knowledge, even hunches are fine. The brainstorm doesn't need to be structured, it is just about making an inventory of the group's knowledge. You might remember from Chapter 2 that new knowledge is linked to old knowledge in the long-term memory, and that for deep learning to occur that old knowledge, 'prior knowledge', needs to be activated. There is a fair amount of evidence that this step really does lead to better retention of facts later. The scribe aims to capture all these thoughts on the board, and a good chairperson will make sure that they manage, by summarising, guiding and preventing everyone from talking at once.

Step 4: Organise ideas

Here the group, often with a lot of help from the scribe, look at the knowledge that they have on the board and try and make sense of it, often by clustering information together. The 'issues' tend to be ignored here, and the information reorganised, and hypotheses are built. This helps link and integrate knowledge across domains, which has been shown to improve retention and recall. Interestingly, even if the hypotheses are wrong, when students later (in step 6) discover that they are wrong, they still learn the right things much better than if they had just read the books without trying to get their thoughts together first.

Step 5: Generating learning objectives

Step 4 will reveal some areas that the group are strong in, that they are sure of, and will also reveal gaps. In our example, the group might well know what diabetes is, and how it is defined and diagnosed, but they might realise that they are unable to explain how glucose causes all the complications of diabetes at the cellular/molecular level, they might be uncertain of what all the possible complications of diabetes are, and they might realise that they are curious about how people adapt to a new diagnosis of diabetes, and what factors help and hinder a positive adaptation. They have therefore generated four learning objectives. They might fine-tune these to be more specific so that everyone is sure what they will be required to answer when they next meet. Often the facilitator (tutor) will have a hidden agenda of some areas that need to be covered for the curriculum.

As a group or as an individual you might generate extra objectives, above and beyond what is expected; perhaps you are interested or curious about something, or perhaps your discussions identified a gap in your knowledge that you need to fill.

Step 6: Self-study

Students study for all objectives on their own. They usually read more widely, but the objectives that they generated guide their study, and at the least they should be able to answer all the objectives that they had agreed as a group. Sources might include books, journal articles and other formal learning materials. More subjective sources might have some value too – expert opinion (including clinicians, patients) and, of course, the Internet – but these sources should be used sparingly. As always, be careful with the Internet – see Chapter 2, p. 33 for some tips on judging the quality of a website. Ideally, you should look at a wide variety of sources and evaluate/triangulate what they say.

Step 7: Reporting back

This step usually happens a few days or a week later. It has the same chair and the same scribe. Often it starts with students going round saying where they found their information. Then each learning objective is taken in turn, and the group explain it, often with one student taking a lead for each objectives. If you have a good facilitator they might ask you sideways questions (perhaps how you would apply your new knowledge to a slightly different situation) to help you elaborate your knowledge, and to help you to see whether you really have understood it as much as you thought you had.

Even though you will have done all your homework on your own, this step helps you learn through teaching/explaining, it also helps you learn through questioning and applying. It allows you to measure the depth and breadth of knowledge that you have learnt against your peers, and is fantastic for motivation.

Making problem-based learning work for you

We have written quite a bit about PBL, and in doing so, we hope that you can see two clear messages that are often misunderstood. First the process is not about generating objectives, it is about maximising subsequent learning and recall. Some institutions actually give the suggested objectives at the beginning of the session, and the students still benefit in terms of relevance, motivation and learning from going through the process. Unfortunately, this approach is rare, and the hidden nature of the objectives often makes them seem the only important thing. (*'We had a great PBL session: we got the objectives out of it in 10 minutes flat'* could be translated as *'We cheated ourselves out of an opportunity for deep learning, and our tutor didn't stop us'.*)

Our second point is simple, everything that you read in the first half of this chapter applies here. Problem-based learning is simply a structured way of going about group work. If you think about the things we covered in the first half of this chapter, and how they influence the way the group works, you will be two-thirds of the way to producing a more productive group.

Study groups

Study groups tend to be groups that students set up themselves in order to learn. Some are more formal than others, but the productive ones tend to follow rules, whether spoken out loud or unwritten. There are usually ground rules about behaviour.

Clinical skills and clinical communication skills

We have discussed how students' own study groups can help development of skills in Chapters 3 and 4. Remember that to learn any skill you need to know how to do it, you need to practise and you need feedback. The two key messages that we want to highlight here are ensuring your learning is active learning, and giving and receiving feedback. Active learning takes two forms: either doing (and you need to practise to learn; however much you watch someone else perform figure skating, you won't be able to do it unless you practise on the ice) or by actively observing. You can learn a lot from watching someone else perform a skill that you are learning – watch attentively and think about what you are learning from doing so. There is no point in being there if you can't see what is going on. Feedback is, of course, essential. Giving constructive feedback (as opposed to destructive feedback, pointless feedback or no feedback) to the other members of your group will help them learn and will keep the group together. Be sure that you are willing to receive feedback from your peers too – ask for it, and pursue it until you get the feedback that you need.

Interprofessional education

As a doctor you will be expected to work closely with other professions – nurses, physiotherapists, dieticians, midwives – the list is a long one. Many medical schools introduce some interprofessional learning, often in small groups, within their curricula to try and help students prepare for interprofessional working later on in life. The aim of such sessions is to help you learn 'with, from and about each other', and on paper they seem like a great idea. In practice it can be touch and go whether such sessions are useful or not.

In her review of interprofessional education (IPE), Della Freeth (2007) argues convincingly that IPE is simply 'a special case of professional education so knowledge about good practise in learning and teaching in a wide range of contexts can be applied directly to IPE', and we agree. To make IPE work, you can apply the contents of this chapter, just as with any other form of group work. If you are aware of roles within the group, of how the group dynamic develops and how you can help it grow, if you pay attention to the behaviours within the group, and are truly curious about other people's point of view, and all the other things that we have covered, then IPE will work well for you.

Summary

Studying, learning and working in a group is essential, and there are many different advantages to doing so. Indeed, some medical school's entire curriculum is based on group work. There are also challenges along the way. In this chapter we have tried to highlight the following factors, which are under your influence, to help you make group work work for you. They apply across any and every form of group work. You won't get it right every time, but we believe strongly that if you are aware of these factors, you reflect on them and invest some perseverance that you will succeed.

- Roles within the group: do you have a good spread? If not, what can you do about it.
- Development of group dynamic: how can you ease the group through the stages to start performing?
- Goals: Are your goals concrete enough? Are they shared? Do they help encourage or discourage collaboration?
- Individual factors: Are you all at a reasonably similar level? Do you appreciate each other's knowledge and skills?
- Behaviours: Does the group ask questions, build links, elaborate knowledge? How about cognitive conflict and debate – is it welcomed? How structured is the process – would more structure help? Are different points of view valued? What does the group do to maximise motivation in its members?

References and further reading

We based much of the educational psychology of collaborative learning on the following papers and texts.

Belbin, R.M. (1981). *Management teams: Why they succeed or fail*. London, Heinemann.

Boxtel, C., van der Linden, J., Kanselaar, G. *et al.* (2000). *Deep Processing in a Collaborative Learning Environment. Social Interaction in Learning and Instruction*: the meaning of discourse for the construction of knowledge. Amsterdam, Pergamom.

Freeth, D. (2007). *Interprofessional Education*. Edinburgh, Association for the Student of Medical Education.

Novak, J.D. (2002). Meaningful learning: the essential factor for conceptual change in limited or inappropriate prepositional hierarchies leading to empowerment of learners. *Science Education* 86: 548–571.

Slavin, R.E. (1996). Research on cooperative learning and achievement: what we know, what we need to know. *Contemporary Educational Psychology* 21: 43–69.

Watkins, B. & Gibson-Sweet, M. (1997). Sailing with Belbin. *Education and Training* 39: 105–110.

Westberg, J. & Jason, H. (1996). *Fostering Learning in Small Groups*: a practical guide. Springer Publishing Company, New York.

If you find you have quite a lot of difficulty working in a group, Stella Cottrell's book gives quite a nice practical guide on simple behaviours that can help build confidence and skills

Cottrell, S. (2003). *The Study Skills Handbook*. Basingstoke, Palgrave Macmillan.

An entry level article on problem-based learning, well worth digging out of the dusty basement of your library is

Schmidt, H.G. (1993). Foundations of problem-based learning: some explanatory notes. *Medical Education* 27: 422–432.

Questions and answers

Q: *I can't work in a group – to be brutally honest, there is no-one I really like in my year, no-one that I really want to spend time with. I am a mature student and all my friends are from outside medical school.*

A: This is a common area of confusion. You do not need to marry people that you study with. They do not need to be your friends. Indeed, sometimes it helps if they are not – especially if you tend to lark about with your friends.

Q: *Everyone in my group keeps shouting each other down, we seem to get nowhere, what can I do?*

A: This might be a normal stage of development of a group, so if it is a one-off, perhaps you should just hang in there. If it has been going on for a while, have you discussed this in the group? Perhaps you could agree some simple ground rules (see above). You might want to seek out some expert advice from a respected, experienced facilitator in the medical school; they are bound to have some tips that will help.

Q: *I hate IPE, what's the point? What could I learn from a nurse?*

A: We know that most major medical errors occur when professions don't communicate effectively and work together; therefore, if you think that there is no point communicating effectively with different professions, then medicine is probably not for you. It is not easy though, it requires a commitment to try and understand someone else's point of view and a large amount of ongoing effort. The desired outcome is excellent patient care through good interprofessional team-working, and with this end in sight, the point becomes clearer.

Q: *Not much group work happens in my medical school, how can I convince people to get a group together?*

A: Lots of people in your year will be feeling the same as you right now. You might want to summarise the start of this chapter (the pros and cons) and talk to those around you. The fact that the whole is greater than the sum of its parts might be a particularly good selling point. Having and communicating a clear structure for the first sessions and a clearly understood objective that people can prepare for will make those first few sessions more likely to succeed – then the ball will be rolling!

Chapter 6 **Developing your academic writing skills**

OVERVIEW

This chapter provides a brief introduction to academic writing. We describe the importance of planning when writing, and highlight some potential pitfalls, particularly with respect to referencing and plagiarism.

Introduction

Writing well is a key skill for a doctor; developing this skill now will stand you in good stead for writing educational materials, research articles, patient information leaflets and even the odd book chapter. Your school will run academic writing courses; you should make an effort to go to one of these courses and apply what you learn as quickly as possible. This section gives a brief introduction to writing an essay, but isn't intended to replace some expert tutoring. You will find whole books on how to write an essay in your library, we reference some in the further reading section of this chapter it would be worthwhile reading one.

Most of the academic writing that you are asked to do at medical school will be set assignments that you write in your own time – either as essays or reflective commentaries (for your portfolio, for example) or other documents. In this chapter we will specifically refer to essays, but the same principles apply to the other forms of academic writing. There are some simple steps to go through to help you construct a winning essay, and in the next couple of pages we have tried to identify one approach.

How to Succeed at Medical School: an essential guide to learning. By Dason Evans and Jo Brown. Published 2009 by Blackwell Publishing, ISBN: 978-1-4051-5139-9.

I really found it difficult to get my thoughts and ideas down on paper in a way that others appreciated. The course that my library ran really helped me to do this.

Jumaane, first-year medical student

Collecting information

If you have read the chapter on note-taking (Chapter 2) you will see lots of techniques that you can use here. You will first either collect your existing notes together and decide what is relevant to the essay, or you will search sources afresh for the essay. Try and do all the searching and reading you need *before* you start the essay, as otherwise you might not realise that the whole focus needs to change until you are halfway through writing. Remember crucially to record sources, so that you can reference them appropriately. Use your own words to make notes, and if you write down any direct quotes, put them in inverted commas in your notes so that you know that you will need to treat them as direct quotes in your essay.

Organise all your information in one place, perhaps as a concept map or MindMap and look for themes that answer the question. Look also for contrasting information that you might highlight as an area of uncertainty.

The message(s)

Decide on what the key points are that you want to cover and decide in what order you would like them to occur. Often there will be one or two key, central messages that you want to get across. In this book, for example, the key messages that we are trying to get across are that the student is the most important person in the learning process; that learning how to learn is an active process which requires deliberate practice and that knowing how you learn (metacognition) results in better outcomes.

Your message may be very clear to you – perhaps you want to argue that drug company advertising should be banned, or perhaps that improving communication skills in doctors will save money in patient care – try and choose an interesting key message, something with a slant. You can then use your essay to explain both sides of the argument, and through this to justify your stance.

Constructing an overview

You might construct your overview using a flowchart, or some sentences or even adapt your concept map from your notes. The patchwork method can also be used, where you make a box for each section of the essay and write key points within each box. You might start the whole process off with a brainstorming session: annotate the session from your reading, organise it in order to answer the question and then further annotate it to make a detailed paragraph plan.

However you go about it, most essays will be divided up into an introduction, a body, conclusions and references. The body might be further subdivided either explicitly using headings (this approach being more common in the sciences) or implicitly using the paragraph contents (more common in the arts).

Make sure that you keep looking back at the question or topic throughout the writing of your essay, and especially at the overview stage (see Figure 6.1). It is easy to get sidetracked into answering a different question to the one that you were given.

> *The trick to writing an essay is to spend plenty of time planning it;*
> *working out what goes where, that makes the writing easy.*
>
> Roger, fourth-year medical student

The paragraphs

You should now have planned the different sections, the things that you want to cover in each section and the order that you wish to cover them. It is time to start writing. In general one idea should go in one paragraph. Often this will form the first sentence of the paragraph, and the rest of the text will elaborate on it (although in this paragraph the key point has arrived only in the third sentence). This rule of thumb will make it easier for the reader to see your main arguments and their justification.

Unfortunately, this approach can come across as a little disjointed, so think about adding a 'link' sentence at the end of one paragraph or at the start of the next. You might, for example, see the first half of the first sentence of this paragraph as a link between these two paragraphs. If your two paragraphs can't link together, then you probably need to go back to your plan and see if you need to rearrange the order that the key points come in, in order to produce a more fluent document.

> *My tutor told me that my paragraphs were all over the place, she showed*
> *me how I could change their order to make a story flow better, and add a*
> *sentence here and there to link them together. I was really impressed at*
> *the finished product!*
>
> Ingrid, intercalated BSc student

Examples of link sentences at the end of a paragraph or start of the next might include:
- 'However, this opinion is not shared by all authors.' Next paragraph: 'Roger Lewis (1993) argues that . . .'

- 'Of course, syphilis is not the only cause of wart-like growths around the anus.' Next paragraph 'Genital warts were first described in . . .'
- '. . . in this way, Wilson felt he had proven the cause of diabetes.' Next paragraph: 'Many other authors at this time also considered that diabetes was caused by an imbalance of the humours . . .'
- Next paragraph: 'These changes have resulted in . . .'

Back to the drawing board
Depending how much of an obsessive planner you are, you might find that new themes or realisations occur to you while you are writing. If this happens you should go back to your plan and see how it fits in; you might need to move your paragraphs around to build a new argument for your new point.

Start at the middle, end with the start
In general, it is useful to end by writing the introduction, which provides the necessary background, relevance and lays out the main arguments, and then finally with the conclusions, which should draw the whole essay together.

Active or passive
One of the dilemmas in academic writing is whether to write it in an active or passive style. Passive styles seem more 'academic' and yet there is considerable evidence that active styles are more readable. Consider the following two introductions:

Communication skills are essential to professional life as a doctor. In this essay I will demonstrate from the literature that poor communication skills result in significant costs, not only in terms of worse patient outcomes and in terms of litigation but also in terms of a social cost to the population as a whole and the trust that it puts in doctors. I will then describe the wide body of evidence that shows that clinical communication skills can be improved through training and will go on to argue for the benefits of mandatory training of doctors in clinical communication skills including its cost-effectiveness.

or

Communication skills are essential to professional life as a doctor. In this paper, the evidence from the literature will be explored to demonstrate that poor communication skills result in significant costs, not only in terms of worse patient outcomes and in terms of litigation but also in terms of a social cost to the population as a whole and the trust that it puts in doctors. A wide body of evidence will be reviewed, showing that clinical communication skills can be improved

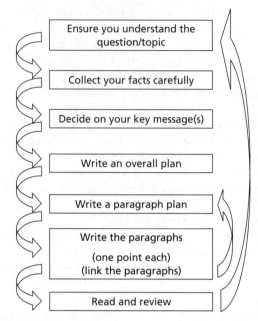

Figure 6.1 Overview of essay writing.

through training and finally a clear argument will be built that the benefits of mandatory training of doctors in clinical communication skills are considerable and would represent a cost-effective intervention.

The first introduction represented an active style ('I will demonstrate'), the second introduction a passive style ('the evidence . . . will be explored'). Experiment with both approaches, and ask your tutors if there is a preferred style in your school. Hopefully the first introduction demonstrates to you that an active style can be used and still make a compelling academic argument.

Plagiarism and referencing

Plagiarism

Plagiarism and referencing is not a focus of the book, but deserves a mention here. If you write down someone else's ideas, you *must* acknowledge them through referencing, otherwise you are passing them off as your ideas, and that is academically dishonest (and is seen by many as equivalent to stealing and lying at the same time). This is why noting down your sources when making notes is so important – so that you know where the ideas came from.

If you directly copy someone's words, it must be *completely* clear that these are their words and not yours; usually you will use quotation marks for this, in addition to referencing. In general it is seen as inappropriate to copy large chunks of text from another source even if you do use quotation marks and references.

Referencing is not only used to demonstrate that you are honest and to acknowledge the 'owner' of the ideas that you use, you should also use references to justify key and controversial points in your essays, and to demonstrate that you have synthesised the literature to inform your points rather than just written down your random opinions.

Note that we suggest that when you are writing an essay, you collect all the information you plan to use in one place first, by making notes in your own words and including some explicit linkage in your notes to the source of information (some people write one large index card for each reference, with the name and detail of the source at the top of the card, others use concept maps with the reference as the root or centre or stem or the map). We then suggest that you try to pick out a message and justify it from these authors. This method makes it easy to avoid plagiarism.

In contrast, imagine the student who writes his or her essay directly from several sources, the books or web pages open in front of him. The temptation will be not to think, not to synthesise and critique the literature, not to build an argument, but rather just to copy out one paragraph from here, one paragraph from there. Not only does the resulting essay look terrible, but the student is suddenly in major trouble for plagiarism.

There are two main forms of referencing: the first is an author–date format when the name and date is inserted in the text as the reference. The proper name for this type of referencing is the Harvard style, and to confuse things there are various different subtypes. Basically, you put the name of the author and the year that they published the paper which you are referencing in the body of the text, and the full details of their paper, book or website reference at the end in alphabetical order. Examples of usage include:

In their paper on preparedness for practice, Evans and colleagues (2004) highlighted feelings of high anxiety in newly qualified doctors.

Anxiety is common in newly qualified doctors (Evans, 2004) . . .

In contrast to Harvard (author–date), the Vancouver approach uses numbers to link to references at the end of the text. Depending on which flavour of Vancouver is being used, the number may be a superscript,[1] or in the text in a round bracket (2) or a square bracket [3]. The *British Medical Journal* uses the superscript approach. Examples include:

In their paper on preparedness for practice, Evans and colleagues[1] high-lighted feelings of high anxiety in newly qualified doctors.

Anxiety is common in newly qualified doctors.[1]

Unfortunately, every different form or flavour of referencing has a slightly different format, especially of the references at the end of your paper. Unless you invest in some software that helps referencing, or your school provides this for free (check with your library, you might be surprised), it is probably best to stick to 'pure Harvard' format for all your essays (the name and date help you remember what you read where) or 'pure Vancouver' if your school required you to use a numbered style. A discussion with your library, or even a simple web search (try the following in a search engine – citation style Harvard) will provide you with all the information that you need to reference appropriately.

Learning more

This book doesn't demonstrate referencing well; it wouldn't rate highly as an academic piece of literature. Most of the text is written from experience and years of working with students, many of them struggling. When we specifically use ideas from other authors we reference explicitly, and when we have turned to several similar texts to make sure that what we are writing is reasonable we cite them as references and further reading. Journal articles are the opposite extreme, ensuring often that every point that they make can be referenced to the wider literature. Have a look at some articles in one of the major journals as examples of referencing, you never know, you might get a taste for reading the journals on a regular basis.

In addition to pointing you toward useful resources, your medical library will run fantastic courses on plagiarism and referencing; go to one early in your course and consider going again a year or two later. These are funda-mental academic skills that will last you a lifetime.

Summary

Although academic writing is becoming a less common activity on medical courses, being able to communicate clearly in a written form is an essential skill for a doctor. Assignments that require academic writing give you a fantastic opportunity to demonstrate your understanding of the complexities around a topic. More is required than just writing, and good preparation by way of searching for information and planning the key messages and detailed structure of the essay before you starting writing will result in much more chance of success.

References and further reading

Your library is likely to have a wide variety of books on essay writing and a huge training resource around referencing and plagiarism. As we have already mentioned, a web search is also likely to be fruitful. You might find some of the following references useful.

Cottrell, S. (2006). *The Exam Skills Handbook:* achieving peak performance. Basingstoke, Palgrave Macmillan.

Evans, M. (2004). *How to Pass Exams Every Time.* Oxford, How To Books.

Lewis, R.S. (1993). *How to Write Essays.* London, National Extension College.

Pears, R. & Shields, G. (2005). *Cite them Right: the essential guide to referencing and plagiarism.* Newcastle, Pear Tree Books.

Questions and answers

Q: If I paraphrase something from the book, then it isn't plagiarism, right?

A: Wrong. If you use someone else's ideas, you must reference them, whether they are their words or not.

Q: I think I have dyslexia, as I find writing essays so difficult – what should I do?

A: Dyslexia is only one of a range of specific learning difficulties, so expert advice would be advised. You should talk this through with your personal tutor and they may well be able to organise for you to have an assessment at your university's learning unit. While this is under way, or even if you do have a diagnosis, you may want to concentrate even harder on planning essays and assignments in the way that we have explained. You might find more visual representations, such a MindMaps and flowcharts, useful in your planning.

Q: My tutor has asked me to write up my project for publication – Help!

A: In addition to the advice in this chapter, have a look at some articles in the journal that you are aiming for to get a feel for the style and structure required. Make a first stab at it (spending particular attention to planning and to referencing) and meet with your tutor. If they have published before then their mentoring will be a great learning experience for you. Don't forget to put them as a co-author on the first draft.

Chapter 7 **Portfolios and reflection**

OVERVIEW

Portfolios are increasingly popular in both undergraduate and postgraduate medical education. Chances are that as a medical student, junior doctor and specialist you will be required to keep a portfolio up to date and you will be assessed on that portfolio. As you will see in this chapter, portfolios are more than just collections of information, they include reflections and often formal reflective commentaries. Students sometimes struggle with the concept of reflection, so we have added a brief section introducing a model for practical reflection.

Introduction

Different institutions use portfolios for different purposes and in different formats, so, not surprisingly, there is often quite a bit of confusion as to what a portfolio is, and more than a little resentment and negative feelings about them. This section aims to clear up some of the mysteries around portfolios, and to help you see how to make a portfolio work in your favour. Because of the wide variety in formats of portfolios we will try and keep most of the advice as generic as possible, with some specific examples to show you how you might apply this advice to your situation. As with the other chapters in this book, you will need to actively engage with the content in order to benefit.

How to Succeed at Medical School: an essential guide to learning. By Dason Evans and Jo Brown. Published 2009 by Blackwell Publishing, ISBN: 978-1-4051-5139-9.

What is a portfolio

A portfolio is a personal collection of information relating to your professional development. More than just containing a record of facts, it is a dynamic and changing document that records and directs your reflections and progress as a medical student and beyond.

What is a portfolio useful for?

From your personal perspective, portfolios are useful for collecting, reflecting and planning. From the perspective of those above you, portfolios are also used for assessing and making judgements.

Imagine that at the start of medical school you buy a big folder and as a front sheet you list the General Medical Council's duties of a doctor (Box 7.1). You buy one of those 12-piece dividers so that you have a section for each of the GMC's six main categories. In each of the six sections you keep information that you gather under that heading. Under 'Provide a good standard of practice and care', for example, you might keep a record of your exam results, under 'Protect and promote the health of patients and the public' you might keep a record of some health promotion teaching that you went to in the first year, and the community health project that you completed in the third year. Imagine that at finals the GMC ask you to demonstrate that you have reached the criteria required for graduation, and you get out your folder (or by then several folders) and show them that you can demonstrate that you fulfil all the duties of a doctor already, your discussions with the GMC would be very easy.

Portfolios tend to be more than a collection of evidence. They tend to include reflections too. Perhaps you will use the spare six sections in your folder to add a commentary or ongoing reflection on the evidence that you submit. What, for example, did you learn from the health promotion teaching that you went to in the first year? In what way will it change your practice? How will you know? What did your last set of exam results tell you? What do you need to do as a result? How will you know that you have made the improvements that you decided on?

You might decide not only to include glowing examples under each of the sections, but also some things that don't go so well. Perhaps in your first year you are disciplined for plagiarism (see Chapter 6) and nearly lose your place in medical school. You might include this under the honesty section and write a reflective commentary on what you learned from the whole experience. Writing a reflective log will help you think about this in a structured way.

Box 7.1 The duties of a doctor registered with the General Medical Council (GMC 2006)

Patients must be able to trust doctors with their lives and health. To justify that trust you must show respect for human life and you must:
- Make the care of your patient your first concern
- Protect and promote the health of patients and the public
- Provide a good standard of practice and care
  - Keep your professional knowledge and skills up to date
  - Recognise and work within the limits of your competence
  - Work with colleagues in the ways that best serve patients' interests
- Treat patients as individuals and respect their dignity
  - Treat patients politely and considerately
  - Respect patients' right to confidentiality
- Work in partnership with patients
  - Listen to patients and respond to their concerns and preferences
  - Give patients the information they want or need in a way they can understand
  - Respect patients' right to reach decisions with you about their treatment and care
  - Support patients in caring for themselves to improve and maintain their health
- Be honest and open and act with integrity
  - Act without delay if you have good reason to believe that you or a colleague may be putting patients at risk
  - Never discriminate unfairly against patients or colleagues
  - Never abuse your patients' trust in you or the public's trust in the profession.

You are personally accountable for your professional practice and must always be prepared to justify your decisions and actions.

By way of helping you plan, imagine that you look through your folder on a regular basis and you decide that under 'Keep your professional knowledge and skills up to date' you cross-reference with the list of skills in one of the GMC's other documents, *Tomorrow's Doctors* (GMC, 2003), and you realise that although they list competence in passing a urethral catheter as a core skill requirement for a new doctor, you haven't done many/any. You therefore find an opportunity to practise in the skills lab and then arrange (with every ounce of charm that you have) to go out on the wards with the urology nurse practitioner, watch him or her in action, and then give it a go on a suitably consenting patient. You keep practising until you are competent and confident. Your portfolio has helped identify a weakness and has helped you plan to address it.

A lot of the learning that you will do in medical school will be through reflections on your interactions with patients in clinical settings. Did things go as expected, or not? Why? What were the strengths and weaknesses of your communication with the patient? Did you miss a key sign on clinical examination? Perhaps you felt that you had failed to build rapport with the patient. A reflective commentary in your portfolio allows you to deconstruct what happened and plan what you might do differently next time, even stimulate you to look some things up.

A portfolio is, therefore, clearly useful to you in terms of collecting evidence, reflecting on and learning from it, and in terms of helping you plan how to fill any gaps in your knowledge or skills. The use of portfolios as an assessment tool is, however, more controversial. Portfolios can clearly be assessed on the quantity and range of evidence that you have collected, but also they can be assessed in terms of the reflections that you have made – do you look like someone who really thinks about what happens (good or bad) and really tries to learn from it?

The real secret of portfolios is to make the portfolio your own. Initially ignore what everyone else tells you, and spend some time thinking about what you want a portfolio for – what will be the focus for you. How would it look? What would be the headings? How often would you look at it? Only after you have an idea of the answers should you go back and look at what the school is asking you to do. Work toward a compromise – something that you own and want, that will also do what the school wants for you too.

The basic structure of a portfolio

There are a thousand different variations on 'portfolio', but depending who you speak to either all or most have a similar structure: all have a list of headings or topics which might be called **goals** or outcomes. These might be as specific as a list of clinical skills that you need to master, or as open-ended as the GMC duties of a doctor in the example above. They might be as impersonal as something your school has set for you, or as personal as something from your heart, perhaps one of your goals might relate to enjoying your social life more.

This list of goals or outcomes is linked to **evidence** that you collect which will reside in folders or sections or under headings. You will probably start with a little evidence from secondary school, perhaps some certificates and exam results, and will build up from there. Of course, one piece of evidence may relate to several goals, so there is usually some indexing or cross-referencing. For example, you may have two goals, one relating to developing a broad anatomy knowledge, the other relating to pursuing a career as a surgeon. Your high mark in a surgical anatomy exam might cross-reference to both goals.

In addition to the evidence, you will need to write some sort of **reflective commentary** on the evidence; this might include reflection on the evidence itself (what did you learn from doing the community health project?), on how this evidence moves you closer to fulfilling your goals (and what gaps are left that still need to be filled) or both. These reflections may generate an **action plan** for change. The concept of 'reflection' is often a puzzle to medical students. Later in this chapter we cover it in more depth.

Special cases: e-portfolios

Paper-based portfolios are reasonably easy to imagine – a folder with sections containing goals, evidence and reflections. e-Portfolios can be more tricky to visualise, but still contain the same structure. An electronic or web-based portfolio has some advantages. It is easy for storage (you don't need to carry around huge folders), and if you choose a web-based version it can be accessible from anywhere in the world, and you can even have different levels of access; you might allow your tutor to see some parts, but perhaps not some of your more personal reflections. For these reasons, in addition to the trend factor, the use of e-portfolios is rapidly expanding in medical schools, and beyond it into postgraduate education.

> IT is my thing, and as I'm webmaster for a student society I thought I had to have an online portfolio, and I found a really good one that was free too. One of my tutors needed some help navigating it, but when I had sat with him and showed him how it works, he thought it was fantastic!
>
> Faruq, fourth-year medical student

You should note some cautions before leaping wholeheartedly into a paper-free portfolio.

- Importantly you should consider the longevity of the portfolio – if your medical school are offering you an e-portfolio, what will happen when you graduate? Will you be able to keep the data and access to it? Imagine that you suddenly have 5 or 6 years' worth of information, all cross-referenced in some nice multidimensional way, not designed to print out, and you have to leave it all behind and try and translate it to some kind of written one or some other electronic version when you leave medical school.
- You might also think about how others will access your portfolio, and if there might be some online access or a useful way of printing out relevant

Goals
Evidence
Reflective commentary
Action plan

Structure of a portfolio

parts. Will it be private and secure enough to keep pranksters away, and yet allow access to those you want?

- The structure of the portfolio is much more open for innovation if all the information is electronic, but be aware that it can rapidly become quite complex and difficult to navigate. You will need to spend time on a regular basis reviewing the structure and adjusting it as necessary.
- Remember that you will still get a lot of evidence in hard copy form – certificates and so forth. You can, perhaps, scan these in if you have access to a scanner, but remember that if it is a high stakes portfolio, you will need to keep the original documents somewhere safe too.

This is not to say anything against online portfolios, but rather to encourage you to think about what you want out of the portfolio and how you should structure it before you spend considerable time, effort and perhaps money on something that turns out not to be as useful as you had imagined.

Perhaps the most exciting aspect of e-portfolios is where they will go next: integration into wikis, blogs (why not keep your reflections as a blog anyway?), social networking sites, directly linking to journals and search engines, and so on. The next few years will be exciting, and you might be a pioneer: be prepared to experiment, and share what works, and especially what doesn't!

Making your portfolio work for you

There are only two rules for making a portfolio useful: you should feel complete ownership of your portfolio, and you should review it regularly. The portfolio should be yours, and yours alone, and you should design it and build it and maintain it for your own benefit. Perhaps you will start one now, using goals that you have generated from this book. One goal might be to develop more effective study skills. You might write a reflective commentary considering how broad and deep your toolkit of study skills currently is, and where you want to develop over the next year. Following on from that you might generate a plan for the next year – to practise using keywords and concept maps for your learning for 3 months, to attend a study skills workshop at your university and to start a study group with some colleagues from medical school. In a couple of months you can see how far you are down that line, if you have collected any evidence, and if it demonstrates progress. You are using this portfolio to drive your own progress.

> *My portfolio is mine, I love it, I spent time making it beautiful and I really enjoy just looking through it, it shows me a map of where I have been and where I am going.*
>
> Mina, third-year medical student

It seems that most humans (not just students) tend to run rather close to deadlines. Non-urgent things are put to the bottom of the pile whereas more urgent things always get put on top. The temptation will be to neglect your portfolio, and you may need to make particular effort not to. Perhaps you could timetable some time every week or fortnight just to file evidence, flick through it, consider where you are (from the evidence) in moving towards your goals (goals), what you have learnt from the evidence and how you are progressing (reflections); you might even write down a paragraph of your thoughts and sometimes you might realise that you need to change direction (action plan). Regular review will mean that your portfolio is always current, always relevant and that it is *alive*. Doing a little, often, will ensure that if anyone wants to see your portfolio, or if you need to dip into it to produce some evidence, no additional effort will be required.

Many of your peers will see portfolios as a nuisance, they will not contribute regularly to them and they will frantically try and complete 12 months' worth of information the night before a portfolio review. Their reflections will be largely fictitious and they will moan about what a 'pointless chore' portfolios are. They are right, *their* portfolio will be pointless, make sure that yours isn't.

Assessment of portfolios

We have already mentioned that there are different approaches to assessing (marking) portfolios. Some institutions just require that a portfolio is kept, others mark on the collection of evidence – perhaps the quantity (consultants are often assessed on the total number of hours of staff development activity that they have completed), or the breadth (are you fulfilling a wide range of goals to become a rounded doctor?). These assessments are relatively easy to design and mark. Some medical schools also mark on the quality of the reflective commentaries. The hope is that this will drive students to reflect often, and result in graduates who can really deconstruct experiences and learn from them. Unfortunately it also drives some students to produce outstanding works of reflective fiction.

If your school marks on the quality of the reflective commentary, it is important to know that they are doing this to encourage you to reflect often. They will be looking for honest accounts, not only of how great you are, but also of where things have gone wrong, what you have learnt from these, how you are planning to improve. If you see the portfolio as belonging to you, and for your benefit, then what is the point of writing fiction, of cheating yourself?

Reflection

What is reflection?

Much has been written about reflection and there are many good books available that examine it in depth. The purpose of this section is to give you an overview and some simple tools to get you started with it quickly.

> *Our minds have two positions: looking out and looking in.*
> (Rinpoche, 1992)

Reflection is the **looking in**, a deep thinking technique that allows us to plan for or analyse events that have already happened and to extract maximum learning from them – a sort of 're-evaluation of experience' (Boud, 2006). Reflection helps to develop an extra level of consciousness or a 'third eye', which allows us to become more aware of our own part or the 'self' in any given situation. Reflective skills are an important part of personal and professional development for all healthcare professionals and some authors argue that it is the main way we effectively learn from experience as adults. Reflecting honestly upon how you learn something or how a particular event has gone is a way of deconstructing experiences and learning from them – a way of learning for real understanding.

> *Reflection was boring, boring, boring until I realised it was just another*
> *way of thinking about what I do and making thinking work for me.*
> Gavin, third-year student

We have already thought about the importance of finding out about your preferred personal learning styles in order to become an effective learner (Chapter 1). Developing reflective skills will also help you to develop your 'third eye' and give you the means to learn from all life events, so that everything is useful and valuable experiences are never wasted.

Some people are natural reflectors, they think about events that have happened, both good and bad and try to work out what went well, what didn't and what their own part in each may have been. For a lot of us however these skills do not come naturally and we have to work at them and actively implement them into our everyday life. Like all new learning skills, it takes a few weeks or months to become comfortable with them, but eventually they become part of what we are and second nature.

The reflective cycle

To get started or consolidate your reflective skills it may be helpful to have a practical model as shown in Figure 7.1.

This can be used as a way of guiding reflection about any event, but as an example of how reflection can be used to think about how you learn, we have mapped a learning experience on to the cycle.

Description: what happened?
'I went to a 1-hour lecture on the functions of the cranial nerves along with my whole year. I came away at the end of it having learned almost nothing and with confused and inadequate notes. There were not enough handouts for everyone and so I didn't even have these to fall back on. The whole lecture seemed like a waste of time for me.'

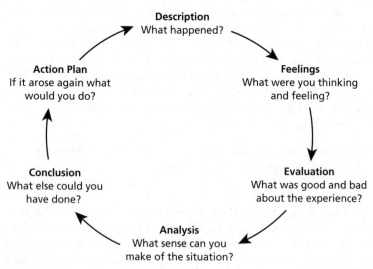

Figure 7.1 The reflective cycle (Gibbs, 1988).

Feelings: what were you thinking and feeling?
'Even before the lecture some of my friends told me that cranial nerves are difficult to learn and yet always come up in exams. The lecturer also began the lecture by saying that this was a difficult subject and that people often fail it in exams. I felt nervous and apprehensive from the beginning and my confidence was low. I don't like lectures at the best of times and often find my mind wanders off and that I don't take good notes. I went home at the end feeling fed up and useless.'

Evaluation: what was good and bad about the experience?
'Lots of bad things, like I still don't know about cranial nerves and probably would fail any exam about them and that I find lectures so difficult. The good thing is that most of the others also find cranial nerves difficult, so I am not alone.'

Analysis: what sense can you make of the situation?
'I know that cranial nerves are important to know about and that I do need to understand them. I need to find a way of learning about them that is right for me. I think that my friends and the lecturer saying that they were difficult had a big influence on my learning and confidence in the lecture. I am more worried about failing exams than learning about cranial nerves!'

Conclusion: what else could you have done?
'I could have prepared for the lecture in advance so that the concepts were not new to me and perhaps made a diagram that could have been fleshed out during the lecture as a way of organising my notes. I think this would have made me more confident. I am going to sit nearer the front next time as it is too easy to let my mind wander when I sit at the back with the other dreamers! I could try recording the lecture to listen to later at home with my notes?'

Action plan: if it arose again what would you do?
'It will arise again as lectures happen frequently. I am determined to be in control in the future and not be influenced by what others say – friends and lecturers have their own motivations and agendas. I also want to discuss lectures in a group to make sure I understand everything and hear what other people have to say. My action plan:
- prepare for lectures to get a head start;
- prepare a rough diagram to shape my notes;
- be aware of my own feelings and how these can impede my learning;
- sit near the front;
- record the lecture;
- consolidate my learning in a group.'

Many people reflect only on the negative or poor experiences, but it is important to reflect on the positive as well. Try applying the reflective cycle to a successful learning experience: establishing what went well and your part in it, will be as valuable as what went wrong.

The reflective cycle can be applied to any situation – professional or private – to help analyse what happened, why and what you felt about it. Try applying it to a situation with friends or family or a patient encounter – it is very adaptable.

> *I find it hard to think about and reflect on difficult times when things have gone wrong because it's like going through the pain again. I do know though that I learn a lot from doing it.*
>
> Femi, fourth-year student

Reflection as a preparation

Reflection can be used as a preparation for learning or for any event (Sully & Dallas, 2005). Consider the following scenario.

You are about to go on a new GP placement tomorrow. You probably have some ideas about what it will be like, particularly as you are a patient registered at a GP practice yourself! It is useful to think about these ideas and thoughts in preparation for the visit. Reflect upon these questions:

- What kind of patients do you think you will be meeting?
- What might be the main challenges to communicating with them?
- What common health problems might they present with?
- Will you be sitting in with the GP or talking to patients on your own?
- Will you be examining any patients?
- How do you feel about the placement?
- Which other healthcare professionals will you be working with?
- How will you record your learning?

Your experience of being a patient will influence how you feel about the GP placement and it will be important to reflect on this. This process may help you to think of strategies for making the placement run smoothly so that it is a rich learning opportunity. After the placement apply the reflective cycle model to analyse how things went and consolidate your learning.

Solo or group reflection?

People find different types of reflection helpful. Once it becomes part of your normal routine, you may find you naturally reflect at certain times of the day, for example on the bus or in the shower. To begin with though you may need to set aside regular times each day to get into the habit. Professor Parveen Kumar (author of one of the leading text books of medicine, past president of the BMA and world-renowned teacher) spends 15 minutes each night writing down a reflective log on what she has learned that day; what better role-model could you follow?

Solo

Some people find writing the best way to reflect and a good way of recording their thoughts so that they are not lost. Throughout history people have kept diaries and these are really just informal reflective journals. A reflective journal can be helpful in returning to a subject to see if things have changed or as a reminder of events or experiences. Written reflection is also a valuable part of any personal and professional development portfolio and can be used to illustrate points or issues you are writing about. Sometimes re-reading a reflective journal can show how much progress you have made or how similar some experiences have been or that a pattern is emerging. Re-reading these after a period of years has elapsed is really interesting, and some authors have even used these as a basis for an autobiography!

Group

Reflecting in a group can be a fascinating way of deconstructing an event or learning experience and will not only provide valuable insight, but also the different perspectives and feelings of everyone else in the group. These can sometimes be so different from your own, that it is a real eye-opener and a way of capturing a much wider view. This sort of group reflective process is sometimes developed further into a critical incident review, when a particular event needs to be analysed and investigated by a whole team as a means of problem solving, and is often used by the NHS and other industries.

Summary

Portfolios and reflections go hand in hand. Portfolios provide a place for you to plan your goals, collect evidence to see that you are reaching your goals, learn from your experiences by reflection and actively plan. Reflection is a structured tool that allows you to learn from experience, and can be used not only in portfolios, but anywhere. We have looked at the definition and applications of reflection in this section and applied these to a learning situation.

- Portfolios are used widely in medical education and come in many different forms.
- Generally they contain goals, evidence, reflective commentaries and action plans.

- Portfolios can really help you be in charge of your own development, which is hugely motivating. Make sure that your portfolio is your own, and review and add to it regularly to make best use of it.
- Reflection is a way of learning about the world.
- Reflection can be used as a tool for thinking about and learning from *any* situation.
- Reflection can be used to prepare for situations.

References and further reading

Boud, D. (2006). The role of work-related learning in developing clinical and communication skills. *CETL Maximising Learning in Practice Conference.* (12.12.06) Barts and the London, Queen Mary's School of Medicine and Dentistry.

General Medical Council (2003). *Tomorrow's Doctors.* London, GMC.

General Medical Council (2006). *Good Medical Practice.* London, GMC.

Gibbs (1988). In: Johns, C. (ed.) *Becoming a Reflective Practitioner.* Oxford, Blackwell Publishing.

Rinpoche, S. (1992*). The Tibetan Book of Living and Dying.* London, Rider.

Sully, P. & Dallas, J. (2005). *Essential Communication Skills for Nursing.* London, Elsevier Mosby.

Questions and answers

Q: My tutor says I don't understand the difference between reflection and description and I don't think I do really?

A: A very common misunderstanding. Any reflective process requires description of the event to some extent as a way of anchoring and capturing what happened. However, this is just stage one of the cycle and you need to go on to think about, evaluate, analyse and plan around the event. Description is just the starting point of reflection.

Q: What is the difference between the words 'reflective' and 'reflexive' as I have seen both used in books?

A: The adjective 'reflexive' describes the act of being a person who reflects e.g. *'The Dalai Lama is a reflexive thinker'* or *'Reflection is a reflexive practice'*.

Chapter 8 **Life–work balance**

OVERVIEW

We hope this chapter will help you to think and plan your life at university and develop a healthy life–work balance. It includes useful ideas about time management and the organisation of study and offers some strategies for recognising and managing stress.

Why is it important?

It may seem odd to devote a whole chapter to life–work balance, but we believe it is so important that it deserves a decent space in this book. Many students we have worked with have found it difficult to achieve a balance between their studies/work and their personal life; in fact, many of our colleagues have similar problems. It may also be a new experience for you to have to balance work and life in a self-directed way, perhaps because teachers, parents or employers have done this for you in the past. What follows are some suggestions for how this might be achieved and also some suggested issues to think about which may be important.

You have chosen to study medicine, which is one of the more demanding university courses and you will certainly have to work hard and devote a reasonable amount of time to it. However, the key word is **reasonable**: study should not normally become overwhelming or all consuming (except perhaps around exam times) and must be balanced against other life activities such as having fun, family/friends, sport, hobbies, etc. Consider what you might think about a doctor who worked all the time and had no 'down time': would you think they had a balanced view of life?

How to Succeed at Medical School: an essential guide to learning. By Dason Evans and Jo Brown. Published 2009 by Blackwell Publishing, ISBN: 978-1-4051-5139-9.

Conversely, if you are the sort of person who has done very little study in the past (perhaps during A-Levels or a previous degree) and have relied on a good memory and cramming before exams to get through, this learning strategy will not work for long at medical school, as there is just too much to remember after a while. Again, consider what you might think about a doctor who studied very little or who spent the minimum amount of time updating their knowledge or skills: would you think they had a balanced view of life, and would you trust them with your own health?

Over an average week, you should aim to be working approximately 1.5 hours each evening, plus 3–4 hours each weekend. This sounds a lot, but is only just over 10 hours per week. These hours may increase around exam times or just before hand-in dates for particular pieces of work, but in the main should not vary greatly. Some people find it easier to work in the library before going home.

> *I stay on after lectures or Case Studies and go to the library around 5.00 pm after a snack. I work until 6.30 and then go home. The rest of the evening is mine then, and I can go out, watch TV, or play computer games without feeling guilty about the work.*
>
> Jonathan, first-year student

As a developing health professional it will be up to you to ensure that there is harmony in your life so that your body, mind and studies are in balance, and if they are not that you are able to ask for help when necessary – more about this later.

Time management

Have you noticed that we all have the same amount of time but that some people use it better than others? Can you think of someone who seems to be organised and always hits deadlines: the chances are that she/he is good at time management. Developing good time management skills can literally *set you free* to concentrate on what really matters in your life by helping to manage all the competing demands on your time in an effective way. Time management skills can be learned and are not necessarily something you are born with, and getting into good time management habits now will serve you for the rest of your life, both professionally and personally.

Ask yourself some questions:

- Do you feel overwhelmed by the amount of studying/work you have to do?
- Do you have difficulty finding lecture notes, handouts, etc., when you need them?
- Are you often behind with paying bills, doing your laundry, renewing library books etc?
- Do you find it difficult to find a clear space to study in your room/flat?
- Do you ever find days or weeks slip by without your having achieved anything concrete?
- Do you spend lots of time making perfect notes that would win the Booker Prize, or record lectures that you never actually listen to again?
- Do you leave study/work until the last minute and then stay up all night to complete it?

If you have answered yes to a few of these, then you probably need to work on your time management skills. It will take practice, but these skills quickly become embedded in everyday life until you forget about them completely.

It hit me when I had missed deadlines for three assignments, owed library fines of over £15.00 and couldn't face the mess in my room anymore that something had to be done – something had to change. I was always trying to catch up with everyone else.

Shobna, second-year student

So, how effective are you at managing your time? Most of us are unaware of the things that take up our time and find it difficult to recall all the things we do each day. To really see what you do with your time, over the next week fill in an activity sheet for each day (Table 8.1), roughly recording the time you do things, what they are and how long they take. At the end of each day put a 'value' (high, medium or low) against each activity.

High-value activities

Are those that are highly essential and must be completed or progressed substantially during the day. They are activities that are directly related to your core study/work objectives and are critical to progress.

Examples: Current Problem-Based Learning or Case-Based Learning, all work which has an imminent deadline, preparation or research for the next day, exam or revision planning, etc.

Medium-value activities

Are less essential activities that it is still preferable, but less critical, to complete or progress substantially during the day. These have to be completed but the time element is less important as the impact on overall study/work objectives is less.

Examples: Deadlines for the following week/month, more long-term projects, research/preparation for medium-term work.

Low-value activities

Are non-essential activities that have a minor impact on your study/work objectives and can be done when time allows or given to someone else.

Examples: Rewriting lecture notes so they are neat or redrawing diagrams until they are perfect; organising the cricket club fixtures for next year; browsing the Internet with no specific search objectives; all projects with no deadlines; interruptions by phone, e-mail or callers.

Table 8.1 Activity sheet

Date			
Time	Activity	Duration	Value

At the end of each day, calculate the total percentage of time you have spent on each category of activity.

- For high-value activities, did you actually achieve what you set out to do?
- If not, what stopped you?
- Could you have achieved more in this category by controlling the low-value activities?
- How could you control low-value activities in the future?

There is a theory in time management called the Pareto 80/20 rule. Vilfredo Pareto was an Italian economist who suggested that 80% of income in Italy ended up in only 20% of the population's pockets! When applied in a time management context this means that without good skills, 80% of our daily activity can generate only 20% of our high-value activities; in other words, we can potentially spend most of our time in producing very little of core importance. Look at your activity sheets (Table 8.1) for the whole week. Are there any patterns emerging? Apply the 80/20 rule. Is it true in your case?

Procrastination

A common cause of putting off important or high value activities is something called **procrastination**, that is putting things off that you should be doing right now. Often procrastinators can't see the difference between urgent activities and important activities. For example:

You have been working on an assignment for the past week and are spending the afternoon writing up your research and findings ready to hand in to your tutor tomorrow. The president of the student union rings to ask you to book a room and refreshments for the meeting that is due to be held that evening in the union building. She has forgotten to do it herself and can't get away from a lecture. You agree to do it even though you know it will take ages and you won't finish your assignment. This is an urgent situation, but it is important? Weigh up the importance of handling in your assignment on time or having a room and refreshments for a meeting. Could you delegate this task?

The MindTools website has a good section on procrastination that you might like to look at as essentially we all suffer from procrastination to some extent, but some people put off important tasks so regularly that it starts to really affect their work. They may work long hours, but concentrate on the wrong tasks. Some common causes of procrastination are:

- *feeling overwhelmed by the task you are supposed to be doing;*
- *feeling unconfident about your ability to do the task, and so getting on with something you* can *do well;*
- *waiting until you feel 'in the mood' to tackle the task;*
- *fearing you will fail (or succeed) at the task;*
- *feeling you don't know how to organise the task;*
- *allowing perfectionism to get in the way ('I can't do the task perfectly, so I won't do it at all').*

(MindTools, 2006)

The way forward with procrastination is to recognise that you are doing it, work out why and then to think of personal strategies for not doing it any more. The reality is that we all have to do things we sometimes find difficult, boring or stressful and it may be helpful to make a daily 'to do' list to help you focus on what needs doing. But also, we all respond well to rewards, so perhaps part of your personal strategy could be the promise of a swim, bubble bath, night out or game of football at the end of a task?

Organisation of your week/month

By planning ahead and organising your week/month in advance you can just concentrate on getting on and not worry that everything is not covered. Table 8.2 shows an example of a timetable designed and used by a second year medical student.

As well as a weekly/monthly plan you will need a diary or personal organiser so that you can book and plan your life in advance.

Organisation of your physical environment

Trying to work in a messy or disorganised environment is always difficult. If you live in an untidy room/flat try at least to keep your desk or working environment clear and organized; your desk is a working machine not a place for storage. Decide on a filing system for your notes and handouts; it really doesn't matter which system you choose as long as it works for you. Get into the habit of reviewing your notes/handouts weekly to refresh your learning, identify any learning gaps and then file them in your system. We think Saturday morning is a good time to do this as it signals the end of the learning week and allows a bit of unpressured time to review, plan and organise. You will revisit these notes many times over the next 4–5 years, so it will save time and energy to organise them right from the beginning. This way you get into the habit of regular review, which means you are revising as you go along and don't have to panic near exam times.

Table 8.2 Weekly timetable planner

21–27 January	Morning	Afternoon	Evening
Monday	PBL tutorial	Lectures	5.00–6.30 study in library 8.00–9.00 yoga
Tuesday	Clinical/communication skills workshops	Work on PBL	5.00–6.30 library – prepare for GP visit 'dermatology'
Wednesday	GP visit	? swim 3.30 dentist	5.00–6.30 library work on PBL and write up reflection on GP visit
Thursday	PBL tutorial	Lectures	5.00–6.30 clinical/ communication skills practice with Michael and Kim
Friday	Expert forum	Lectures	Pizza and a film
Saturday	Lie in 10.00–12.00 go over the week's lecture notes and PBL notes, file them	Washing, cooking, shopping, etc.	
Sunday	Lie in	4.00–5.30 prepare for next week	

Stress management

With a good balance of work and play in your life there shouldn't be too much stress to manage, particularly if you are organising your time effectively. Once you have a good time management plan going things tend to run smoothly in the main. Stress is part of modern life and to some extent is good for us, helping and challenging us to perform at a high level. Stress levels fluctuate depending on what we are doing and we need to be aware of them so that we can intervene if they get too high. There are many causes of stress:

- exams
- deadlines
- presentations
- money
- relationships

- health
- family, etc.

It might be helpful to look at the physical response our bodies have to stress.

The fight/flight response (Figure 8.1)

This primitive response was vital in the days when physical danger from wild animals and hostile tribes required us to either fight or run away from the danger. Of course dangers still exist in modern society, and in order to cope with them our bodies continue to produce adrenalin to support the fight/flight response. Table 8.3 shows some of the physical changes that take place during this process.

Stress and anxiety can trigger exactly the same fight/flight response in our bodies, but unlike being chased by a bull, there is no natural end to the response and so the adrenalin continues to circulate in our bodies triggering a physical response. The **stress/anxiety cycle** works as in Figure 8.2.

This circular motion continues unless we can break into the stress/anxiety cycle to control the physical response, and this can be done very simply by **deep breathing** and **relaxation**. By slowing down our breathing and taking in deeper breaths, we can interfere with the messages being sent to the brain and therefore control the fight/flight reflex. Look at the different physical effects stress and relaxation has on us (Table 8.4).

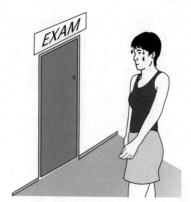

Figure 8.1 The stressed student demonstrates the fight/flight response.

Table 8.3 Physical changes taking place when stressed

Increased activity	Decreased activity
• Pupils dilate • Circulation increases blood supply to brain, muscles and limbs • Heart beats quicker and harder: coronary arteries dilate • Blood pressure rises • Lungs take in more oxygen and carbon dioxide • Liver releases extra sugar for energy • Muscles tense for action • Sweating increases to aid heat loss blood clotting ability increases • Adrenal glands secrete adrenalin	• Digestion slows down or stops: stomach and small intestines reduce activity • Mouth goes dry: constriction of blood vessels in salivary glands • Kidney, large intestine and bladder slow down • Immune responses decrease • Sphincter muscles close to prevent urination and defecation

Danger/threat which is real or imagined

Brain continues to send messages to respiratory organs to prepare for action

Message sent to brain to prepare to run

Shallow, quick breathing develops

Release of too much carbon dioxide so that the brain believes there is a threat

Figure 8.2 The stress/anxiety cycle.

Table 8.4 The different physical responses of stress and relaxation

Stress response		Relaxation response
Up	Heart rate	Down
Up	Blood pressure	Down
Up	Breathing rate	Down
Up	Muscle tension	Down
Up	Sweating	Down
Up	State of mental arousal	Down
Up	Adrenalin flow	Down

So deep, slow breathing and periods of relaxation are important for all of us and we need to practise how to do them well. Relaxation needs to happen regularly during the day and here is a simple exercise to try.

EXERCISE

- You can relax sitting in a chair, on the bus/train or lying down. It can take just 5 minutes. Make sure you are feeling warm.

- Close your eyes and think consciously about your breathing. Take three deep in-breaths, holding them in for a few seconds before exhaling. Make sure you empty your lungs of stale air completely.

- Think about your body systematically, starting with your feet and working up to your head and neck – consciously feel and relax each part you think about, until all of you is relaxed and heavy. Pay particular attention to your shoulders, jaw, around your eyes and forehead.

- Now in your mind, go to a beautiful or favourite place where you have felt relaxed and happy and just imagine yourself there for a few minutes.

- When you are ready, come back to where you are and become aware again of your surroundings and the sounds around you. You should feel calm, relaxed and less tense.

Interestingly, feeling relaxed and calm helps us to access memory and language skills, concentrate better, study in more depth and retain what we learn, so regular relaxation helps us with study as well as probably helping us to live a longer life!

Every time I even thought about exams I started to feel ill, my mouth and throat closed up and my stomach churned until I though I would be sick. The student counsellor recommended I take up Yoga so that I could learn to relax and control my breathing even in really stressful situations. I didn't take it seriously at first, but when I got into it I felt a bit more confident about not losing it in exams

Sam, first-year student

Seeking help

As we mentioned earlier in this chapter, sometimes sensible balances, regular study and relaxation are not the only answers because the problems are different or deeper and you may need help from someone else. From time to time we all need to call on our GP, Counselling Service or Student Welfare organisation but the important issue here is that as a developing health professional you feel able to ask for help if life feels miserable or overwhelming for whatever reason. There is a difference between feeling anxious sometimes and feeling anxious *all* the time, or between feeling sad occasionally and feeling sad *most* of the time. Medical students and doctors can lead pretty stressful lives sometimes and it really is vital to ask for help when you need it. Indeed the mark of a competent professional is the ability to seek help when necessary.

Relaxation tips from students

'I run around the block as fast as I can to relieve stress – it works!'

'Planning and cooking a meal helps me to relax.'

'Playing computer games is my best stress buster – I have to watch this though as hours can pass unnoticed.'

'The usual stuff really, bath, bed, good book or TV.'

'I watch old episodes of Star Trek – very relaxing.'

'Going to the gym followed by a sauna.'

'If I wake up at night feeling stressed, I get up, write down what is worrying me and any thoughts or solutions I am thinking about and then go back to sleep. I know it is then all written down and not lost!'

'A glass of wine with friends can put things in perspective.'

Summary

We have looked at the importance of achieving a balance between life and work in this section and suggested some strategies for achieving it. We have looked at planning study and leisure and recognising procrastination as well as seeing the physical effects of stress and its management. We ended with relaxation tips from students.

- Achieving a balance between work and life is essential for the whole of professional life.
- Analyse how you use your time to see if you are effective.
- Planning and organising your time literally sets you free.
- Make a study plan each week/month and stick to it.

References and further reading

MindTools (2006) *Mind Tools Activity Log: essential skills for an excellent career.* www.mindtools.com/rs/ActivityLog.

Questions and answers

Q: I already had a degree when I started at medical school and thought that I knew how much time to devote to study. But, my usual two or three evenings per week are just not enough, and I am only in the first year!'

A: Medicine does require more hours of study than most other degrees and because it covers such a diverse array of subjects needs a systematic approach. Ten hours a week of well planned study is the average, with an effective filing system to manage information and notes. As you progress on the course the nature of the study may change somewhat, particularly when you enter the clinical environment and are learning from patients.

Q: I seem to spend every evening studying although my flatmates go out and seem to do OK in exams. Maybe I am not as bright as them?'

A: This is a common concern and to a certain extent we all worry that we are not clever or good enough. Interestingly we have almost never found this to be the case when working with students. However, anxiety can often get in the way of effective study and the key really is the quality of study rather than the quantity, although we all have individual study habits. It may be helpful to look at your flatmates' study techniques to discover how they are able to balance their lives and still be successful in exams. See Chapter 2: this discusses methods for effective study.

Q: I have to work on Saturdays and one evening during the week to support myself at medical school. The work seems to pile up and I never seem to finish.

A: It is very difficult to have a job whilst you are studying medicine as the course is so demanding, particularly when you reach the clinical years and may need to do on-calls or stay on to see a particular patient or procedure. You will need to develop excellent time management skills to balance all the demands and develop good study plans so that every hour of study really counts. Remember however that many people do need to work to support themselves and indeed many medical students have children to care for as well as studying. Be careful to ensure you are eating and sleeping properly and have one night a week when you can completely relax.

Q: If I tell my tutor that I'm struggling, won't it count against me?

A: Your tutors are involved in education because they want to help students to do well. Over the years they have seen hundreds of struggling students and will be able to offer you good advice and support. Imagine you perform badly in an exam, if the medical school knows that you have identified a problem and that you are working to overcome it, this can only work in your favour.

Chapter 9 **Revision**

OVERVIEW

This chapter will help you plan for revision in a realistic way and will suggest some techniques that may be helpful for revising knowledge and skills. We have also collected general experiences and tips from medical students and share them here. We end as usual with commonly asked questions.

What is revision?

At a basic level, revision is a systematic way of reminding yourself of what you have learned in preparation for a written or practical exam. So much has been written in the last decade about the best ways to revise, and the most efficient techniques for committing things to memory, that choosing a personal path for revision may be confusing with so many choices available. Remember that you are already adept at passing exams because you have successfully gained GCSEs, A-levels and perhaps a degree. As you already know, revision isn't rocket science, but it is a necessary part of your learning repertoire, and like anything else revision skills can be made more effective.

We have mentioned before the importance of revising right from the beginning of the course rather than leaving things to the last minute. This way, you build your knowledge, understanding and skills gradually and systematically over time, which will increase your confidence level. If you have managed to review and organise your notes, lecture handouts, articles, etc., each week into a logical filing system, then you are already halfway there. You will have been revising as you went along and now it will simply be a matter of refreshing your understanding and perhaps getting in some practice for any practical exams.

How to Succeed at Medical School: an essential guide to learning. By Dason Evans and Jo Brown. Published 2009 by Blackwell Publishing, ISBN: 978-1-4051-5139-9.

An important thought we would like you to hold in your mind whenever you are revising is to imagine that you are the examiner setting a question on this topic.

- What understanding would you want to test?
- What question would you ask to test it?

Having this overview always present in your mind will help you to see the knowledge and skills you have acquired from an assessment perspective and will help you to visualise the questions and tasks that you may be asked in an exam.

What kind of techniques?

So, what kind of revision techniques will work for you? Do you learn well from books? Is it better for you to discuss what you learn in a group? Are you a visual learner who enjoys diagrams or graphic representation of things? As with all learning, we are all unique and do things in different ways, but interestingly research has shown:

> We remember 20% of what we read
> We remember 30% of what we hear
> We remember 40% of what we see
> We remember 50% of what we say
> We remember 60% of what we do
> We remember 90% of what we read, see, hear, say and do
> (Turner, 2007)

So, a mixture of revision methods may be useful.

Draw up a plan

It is vital to spend a few hours drawing up a comprehensive revision plan right at the start. Perhaps have one timetable for each week, decide upon the focus for that week and then break this down for each day, scheduling how long you will spend revising each topic. Remember to factor in time to eat, relax and have a period of exercise each day to counteract periods of inactivity – a long walk or a swim. Draw up revision into blocks of 1.5 hours with 30-minute gaps between to stretch your legs and get a drink. So, each revision block lasts 2 hours and you could aim to do three or four blocks for each full day, or maybe one if it is an evening session. Factor in at least two periods each week when you will revise with others in a group.

Providing you have made a comprehensive plan that covers the subjects to be revised and you stick to it, you can stop worrying about whether everything will be covered (Table 9.1).

Table 9.1 A sample revision timetable from a third-year student revising the heart

Day/date	AM	PM	Evening
Monday 18 Jan	Anatomy of heart	Physiology of heart	5.00–7.00 gym and supper 7.00–9.00 draw rough anatomy, create consolidate diagrams, self-testing
Tuesday 19 Jan	Heart failure: main presentation	Heart failure: treatment and management	5.00–6.30 supper and walk 6.30–8.30 consolidation, self-testing
Wednesday 20 Jan	Myocardial infarction: main presentation	Myocardial infarction: treatment and management	6.00–7.00 supper Revising heart failure and myocardial infarction with Chris
Thursday 21 Jan	Group revision on whole topic	Revise topics identified in group revision	6.00–8.00 supper and gym Prepare for practical session tomorrow
Friday 22 Jan	Group work practising history of chest pain, examining the chest, feedback	Reflect on group practise: identify gaps and weaknesses	Epidemiology of heart disease
Saturday 23 Jan	Day off	Day off	Day off
Sunday 24 Jan	Lie in	Consolidate all topics from this week. Fine tune, finishing touches to notes. Put away files and books not needed any longer	Plan for next week's revision. Get out notes, appropriate books, etc.

Three student commentaries on revision

I like to review all my (fairly extensive) notes and handouts at the end of each week and file them into module files. I then revise one module at a time in the weeks before an exam. It takes me about 4 weeks to cover each module. I don't write out special revision notes as this would be

duplicating the work. I make every set of notes work for me, so it's worth getting them right from the start. I prefer revising on my own, but sometimes get together with others to practise clinical skills. I like working with other people when I don't understand something. I also like reading a wide range of text books to make sure I've got my head around everything. I revise about 5 nights a week before exams but keep weekends free for other things.

Rachel, second-year graduate student

We set up a 'learning objectives' revision group where we look at the learning objectives for all our PBLs [problem-based learning]and clinical placements and then make sure we have covered everything, that way there are no surprises in exams. Our revision group works like a PBL group – all of us decide which aspects of a subject to find out about and we share in a group our findings. We have a scribe who records everything but I make my own notes and diagrams, which I condense into a final revision summary. I tend to start revising 8 weeks before an exam and don't do much else. I revise on most days and tend to put my life on hold.

Kris, third-year student

Because I have two young children, it's difficult to get a routine going for revision. I try to keep my notes in order so that the course doesn't get out of control and everything is kept in a filing cabinet out of the way of the children. I often get up at 5.00 am to work as I am good in the mornings. My husband has the children all day on Saturday so I have a good stretch of time to revise in – I always go to the library though as it's quiet. I find that I can revise in a really focused way in quite small amounts of time (20 minutes) and I tend to do this throughout the day. I think having the children has taught me not to waste a minute.

Lea, first-year graduate student

Organise your space

We talk in Chapter 8 about organising your desk or learning space. For the purposes of revision, however, we recommend a more radical reorganisation of your life! The reason for this is to minimise all distractions so that you can really concentrate on revising. So, before getting down to the work some preparation is necessary:

- clean your flat or room
- sort out and put things away
- change the bed
- organise your desk

- stock up on healthy food and snacks
- do the laundry
- tell everyone you are about to start revising
- make a 'do not disturb' notice for your door.

Think about 'known distracters': are there some things that always tend to distract you. Perhaps telephone calls, instant messaging on your computer or switching the TV on for a second when you have a break only to find yourself sat in front of it 2 hours later? Plan how to avoid these; perhaps switch off your phone, unplug from the Internet, put a towel over the TV.

If you live in a place where it is not possible to study in a quiet environment without interruption, then you will need to revise in the library or other room at college. Tutors will be able to help you organise this.

During A levels I was always able to revise everything really quickly just before exams but this didn't work for me at med school. I had to retake my second year because I failed exams on two occasions and had to learn a different way of studying for deep understanding. I think I was a late starter!

Joel, fourth year student

Revising knowledge

An important thing for you to know is that just copying out notes from a book or handout will not help you understand or remember them. You need to interpret them and put them into your own words, perhaps by paraphrasing them or converting them into a MindMap or flow chart (see Chapter 2). This is the difference between **note taking** or recording the factual content of say, a lecture and **note making** which includes your analysis and interpretation of the information (Evans, 2004). Exams in the main test your understanding of a topic, not your ability to just memorise it, although there may be a small amount of information that you will need to just remember. After paraphrasing your notes, turn them over and see what you can remember and write out again. You will now understand how useful the advice in Chapter 2 is. If you use Cornell notes, or some of the other techniques that we discussed such as writing questions as you go along, this process will be much easier for you. Try revisiting your notes again in a week's time to see how much you have retained. Perhaps record your notes and try listening to them as you walk around. Pretend you are giving a lecture about this topic; what would you say and how would you organise it?

You probably already use revision cards, Post-it notes, coloured highlighter pens and mnemonics such as:

- site
- onset
- character
- radiation
- associated symptoms
- timing
- exacerbating and relieving factors
- severity,

a useful basic mnemonic when asking a patient about pain. All of these are helpful tools.

> *I made a batch of revision cards which I carried about with me and looked at when I had slack time, like on the train. I find it easier to revise in short bursts rather than a long session*
>
> Alice, first-year student

It is often said that the best way to learn something is to teach it and you may like to do this in a learning group, with everyone taking turns at teaching a topic. This works on two levels; first, it shares some of the work of the revision, but it also allows you to test your level of understanding of a topic against your peers. Are you more or less on a level with the others or are you revising a topic in too great a depth? Are you revising a good breadth or overview of a topic, but not understanding enough of the detail? Learning with others will give you a good gauge of breadth and depth.

You may like to look at past papers to get an idea of what has gone before and how questions are written and presented. Try doing some of these papers and timing yourself. Get familiar with the types of question you may be asked such as:

- extended matching questions
- multiple choice questions
- short answer questions
- best answer questions.

Being familiar with the format of the question will allow you to practise and will boost your performance. A really useful exercise is to get a group of people to sit a past paper together. Compare the results and decide upon a model answer for each question. How did others in the group tackle the question style? Chapters 10 and 11 look at common question styles and approaches to managing them in more depth.

Revising clinical and communication skills

You may already be familiar with a range of written exam formats from your previous study, but the main way that clinical and communication skills are tested at medical school is in an Objective Structured Clinical Examination

(OSCE), a practical exam that may be less familiar. In an OSCE, a large room is divided into a number of 'stations', each one focused on a different task. Each station may contain a model, image, simulated patient or real patient and an examiner and you will be asked to carry out a task in 5–10 minutes before a bell rings and you move on to the next station. The examiner will mark you on a range of items connected with the task. The great thing about OSCEs is that although they can be nerve wracking, you get a broad range of opinion about your competency, for if there are say 17 stations in the OSCE, then 17 examiners assess you.

In stark contrast to revising knowledge, clinical and communication skills need to be actively revised in pairs or in a group, with **feedback**. You will probably have already covered the main skills to be revised during your course, but these must be practised, practised, practised!

We suggested earlier that just like any other sort of revision, clinical and communication skills should be practised informally on a weekly basis with your peers, although remember that revision cannot replace real experiences, but hopefully that message was clear in Chapters 3 and 4. It is also helpful if this revision is integrated. The following exercise suggests about how this can be organised:

EXERCISE: AN INTEGRATED APPROACH TO REVISING CLINICAL AND COMMUNICATION SKILLS

- Decide as a learning group on a topic – say asthma
- The whole group revises the knowledge base for asthma, makes notes, diagrams, collects articles, etc.
- One member of the group writes a 'patient scenario' or role play that includes the clinical details of asthma and joins these with relevant psychosocial issues the patient may be experiencing.
- One person plays the 'patient' and the group take it in turns to interview them about their asthma – don't forget to give each other feedback on the interview, perhaps dividing it into 'content' (the information that was gathered) and 'process' (the communication skills used to elicit the information). Use the checklist of communication skills (Chapter 4).
- The group has also looked at skills books and skills handouts on examining the chest, and together you agree on a 'gold standard' for doing this and draw up a checklist.
- A group member agrees to have their chest examined and you take it in turns to examine each other using your gold standard checklist and not forgetting to give feedback.
- Don't forget to have your 'examiner's' hat on! If you were writing an OSCE station about asthma, what items would you test and what would you give marks for? We cover OSCEs in more depth in Chapter 11.

*It was hard to connect all the things we had learned in lectures and
PBLs [problem-based learning] to skills. I tried to learn it all from books
because I'm OK at that, but in the end I realised it was about practising
the skills with real people. Once I started doing that I got
the hang of things.*

Ryan, second-year student

Of course, the very best way to revise clinical and communication skills
is with real patients, but you may not have reached that stage of the course
yet, and so working in a group with colleagues and any simulation models/
equipment your medical school may have is a good substitute.

The connection between smell and memory

This connection has been well known for many years, but research at the
University of Northumbria found that smelling rosemary oil 'produced a
significant enhancement of performance for overall quality of memory'
(Moss *et al.*, 2003) in healthy adults. This connection can be put to good use
in revision. Try this:
- buy an aromatherapy oil burner and some rosemary oil (don't use
  rosemary oil if you are pregnant);
- burn the oil whenever you are revising, but never at any other time;
- just before going into the exam, put a few drops of rosemary oil on a tissue
  (never directly on to your skin) and smell it at regular intervals during
  the exam.

Conversely, the same research found that lavender oil significantly decreased
memory and performance, so if you are finding it difficult to switch off after
revision and sleep, you could try using lavender on your pillow!

General hints and tips

These have been gathered from many people and sources, but particularly
from medical students who found them helpful.
- Make a 'do not disturb' notice for your door. Tell friends and family that
  you are revising and get their help. Stick your revision timetable on the
  outside of your door so that people can see what you are doing.
- Turn off your phone for regular periods when you are revising. Tell people
  that you are going to do this.
- Eat and drink regularly. There is a well-known connection between healthy
  food eaten at regular intervals and learning performance. Eat breakfast and

have snacks such as bananas, sesame seeds, tuna fish, dried fruit, avocados, nuts, etc. Drink plenty of water.

- Exercise every day to combat stress and inactivity. It will help you sleep.
- Gentle music helps some people revise and you can even buy specially designed CDs in music shops if you feel so inclined. TV, however, *never helps* – turn it off.
- Cross off each topic you revise from your revision timetable; this is deeply satisfying and charts your progress.
- Go to bed at a reasonable time and get enough sleep. Revising into the night can be counterproductive.
- Try visualising yourself entering the exam feeling calm, happy and in control. Try to imagine what the room will look like and see yourself during the exam calmly writing or performing a task in an OSCE station. Keep this positive image in your head.

What if I fail?

Most of us fail something in our lives and miserable as that can feel, failing an exam will probably make you a better doctor. Why? Because you will develop strategies to overcome the failure and pass re-take exams and you will have gained valuable experience and insight into what it feels like to fail, which in turn will develop your empathic skills.

Failing an exam is not the end of the world, even if it feels like it at the time, and most medical schools will be able to offer you some help and support in preparing for a re-take exam or repeating part of the course. Get as much feedback as you can about why you have failed so that you can identify your strengths and weaknesses and get together with any others who have also failed to develop a plan and form a learning group to prepare for what comes next.

Try talking to students in the years above you about their revision techniques and tips; often they will have developed sophisticated strategies and there is never any point reinventing the wheel! Conversely though, no one strategy fits everyone and you will need to design revision around your own strengths and weaknesses and learning style.

Summary

In this section we have looked at what revision is and what it isn't. We have highlighted the differences between revising knowledge and skills and looked at the connection between smell and memory. We have highlighted the practical implications of drawing up a good revision plan and managing your revision space and have seen examples of revision strategies from three students and some suggestions for integrated revision in a group.

- View the subject you are revising from an examiner perspective.
- Exams test understanding and not memory.
- Revise from the beginning of the course.
- Make a good revision plan and stick to it.
- People revise in a variety of effective ways.
- Spend some time revising in a group.

References and further reading

Evans, M. (2004). *How To Pass Exams Every Time*. Oxford, How To Books Ltd.

Moss, M., Cook, J., Wesnes, K., Duckett, P. *et al.* (2003). Aromas of rosemary and lavender essential oils differentially affect cognition and mood in healthy adults. *International Journal of Neuroscience* 113: 15–38.

Turner, L.K. (2007). Revision techniques, *Business Studies*. Woodside High School, Wood Green, London.

Frequently asked questions

Q: I seem to spend hours revising but can't remember anything in the exam.

A: A common problem that may be due to poor revision technique. You may spend hours revising, but is it quality revision? Have you made a timetable, allocated topics to blocks of time, paraphrased your notes, and shared revision with a group? It really is about the quality of the revision and not the quantity. Beginning your revision in good time will also increase your confidence because you will know you have everything covered.

Q: I seem to panic just before going into an exam.

A: Exams can be very stressful and most people feel a bit panicky at the start. Remember that this panic will cause a 'fight or flight' reaction. Go through the breathing and relaxation techniques suggested in Chapter 8 and think about a more long-term solution such as yoga. If this becomes a really big problem for you, then you need to seek help from your counselling service who may be able to help you develop individual strategies to combat your panic.

Q: I lost a load of my revision notes on the bus.

A: This bad luck can be turned into a really good revision tool! Ask to borrow other people's notes, look at the books to check the content, paraphrase them into something that makes sense to you. Compare revision notes for depth and breadth, present what you have learned in a group. By doing all of this you are actively revising and may even revise more effectively this way!

Q: I never know how soon to start revising before an exam.

A: I hope that we have convinced you that revision is something you should be doing as you go along every week, and that the last few weeks before an exam should be a time for fine-tuning and consolidation, as you won't be able to cram a year of learning into 5 weeks! A few weeks before the exam, draw up a revision timetable so that you can review and remind yourself of what you have learned. Leave plenty of time so things are not rushed and there is time to cover things in enough detail.

Chapter 10 **Exam technique: general rules**

OVERVIEW

This chapter provides an overview of the general rules for any exam. Many of these are simple, and yet we know from many students that they can be neglected. You will read most of this chapter quickly, and we suspect that it will make a lot of sense. You might want to read it again a week or two before you sit your first set of exams, perhaps subsequent sets of exams too.

In Chapter 11, we shall try and apply these general principles to the specific exams that you are likely to come across in your time at medical school.

Introduction

This chapter brings bad news and good news. The bad news is that contrary to popular belief, cunning exam technique will not allow you to pass exams at medical school without doing any work. The good news, however, is that appropriate exam technique will help you demonstrate what you know to your advantage.

Preparing for the exam

Knowing the format and rules of the exam

Students who struggle often tell us: 'I didn't know what to expect from the exam'. It might seem obvious, but you should invest some time **finding out about the exam**, including it's structure and format. How many questions, how much time, what sort of questions will there be? All this information is crucial to your preparation. There will be formal information such as exam

How to Succeed at Medical School: an essential guide to learning. By Dason Evans and Jo Brown. Published 2009 by Blackwell Publishing, ISBN: 978-1-4051-5139-9.

briefings and written information, but don't forget the informal information including impressions from students in the year above: 'There was much more anatomy than I was expecting' or 'I didn't realise that the questions would expect us to explain pathology in terms of what we knew of anatomy and physiology' will be invaluable to you.

One word of warning though, remember that these are rather subjective judgements. At one institution we know, performance in the third year exams would oscillate: one year many students would fail the clinical exam, and few the written; these students would then pass on the message that the clinical exam was really hard and 'no-one ever failed the written' and the following year students would come well prepared for the clinicals, but poorly prepared for the writtens. This caused a rather predictable 2-year cycle. You might, therefore, try and speak to students in several years above you and try and build a consensus on their advice. Think about useful questions that you could ask, such as:

- What exactly happened in the exam?
- What was different from you expected?
- If you were doing the exam again, what would you do differently in your preparation?

If you know the format of the exam, you can practise some **mock exams**. Perhaps you will use past papers, questions from books or the Internet or even write your own (see our previous discussions about writing questions as you study in Chapter 2). As we discussed in our Chapter 9, perform under exam conditions and especially under exam timings. Use these practice papers as a chance to practise technique, and also as a diagnostic tool. If you get a question wrong, **do not** just memorise the right answer, but rather go back and revise that area again. Imagine that you get a question on one of the treatments of diabetes wrong; this probably means that you need to look at all the treatments of diabetes again, perhaps even that you need to ensure that you understand the whole of diabetes.

Extenuating circumstances

Every institution has an **extenuating circumstances** policy. You may not wish to think about this, but imagine that something terrible happens to you around the time of an exam: perhaps a family member falls ill or water starts pouring into your flat and you have to camp out on a friend's floor. In these cases your institution might take these circumstances into account when looking at your results. Examples might include (different for each institution):

- If you don't turn up for an exam, this is usually counted as a fail, reducing the number of further attempts that you can have at this exam, and placing a bit of a black mark on your record. If you have good reason, the exam board might agree to make the next sitting of the exam that you do count as a 'first sit'.

• If something terrible has happened to you around the time of the exam, and your result comes out at just a very little below the pass mark, the exam board might look at your extenuating circumstances and agree that they prevented you from demonstrating your true level on the day of the exam.

True to form, when things go wrong, the last thing you will want to do is try and find out the regulations and paperwork for extenuating circumstances. Get these papers together well before the exam and keep them somewhere safe; hopefully you will not need them, but you or a friend might be grateful for your preparation one day.

While talking about extenuating circumstances, we ought to also highlight a few points. First, exam boards really aren't impressed with frivolous claims: if your hamster died 2 months before the exam, they are really unlikely to want to hear about it. They only want to know if there is a valid reason that your performance *on the day* did not reflect your knowledge and skills. Similarly, if you have a long-standing problem that has affected your work, perhaps your recurrent admissions to hospital with asthma and chest infections has meant that you missed most of the teaching this year, and then you fail the exam, they might surmise that you didn't have the knowledge and skills required for you to pass the exam because of all the time you lost, and so you should, indeed, have failed. If you were in A&E all night the night before the exam with an asthma attack, and wheezed your way through the exam after a sleepless night, they might, instead, surmise that it would be reasonable for your mark to be a little higher.

> The university learning support unit thought that I might have dyslexia, they referred me to an educational psychologist who confirmed it and wrote a report for the exams office. I now have extra time in written exams, and feel far less stressed.
>
> Jamie, second-year medical student

Clearly, any claim you make will need to be honest and you will need to be able to provide written evidence to back up your claim. Whatever happens don't lie. If things are going wrong for you in the lead up to the exams, just as at any other time, don't forget that the school would rather know about it sooner than later, and that people are in place to help and support you (see Chapter 8). Most extenuating circumstances policies only work if you make the school aware of your difficulties before the exam, and *never* after the results are out.

Learning from the past

The final thing to consider before the exam is your **previous experience.** How have previous exams gone? Where are your strengths and weaknesses? If you often get too nervous before an exam you should plan months in advance what you can do about this (see next section and Chapter 8). Similarly if you find a certain format of exam particularly challenging, then you should actively plan how to address this before the exams. Some tips in the following sections might help, as will various courses that your school will run. Students who say 'it's funny, but I never do well in multiple choice exams' don't get much sympathy!

Dealing with nerves

Everyone gets nervous before an exam. This is normal, and indeed a bit of adrenaline probably helps you perform better. If you have been following the advice in this book then you should have learnt the content of the course and revised it as you have gone along, using deep techniques that ensured understanding and effective recall (Chapter 2), you will have revised well (Chapter 9), and you can relax in the knowledge that you are well prepared.

Of course some people get very nervous at exam time, and in addition to the advice that we gave in Chapter 9 (revision) there are some simple tips to follow on the day.

- **Be early for the exam** – the last thing you want to feel on the day is the panic that you might not make it in time for the exam. Aim to arrive at least half an hour (more if you are travelling a distance to get there) before the start of the exam.
- **Speak only to people who will make you feel good about the exam** – this advice from Stella Cottrell (2006) is important. Louise's advice below gives a good example of learning from experience.

I failed my first year exams because I was too nervous – I turned up and stood outside the exam hall with all my friends, and listening to them talk about all the things that they had learned made me panic, and in the exam all I could do was think that I hadn't prepared enough, rather than the questions in front of me.
Every exam I have taken since then, I have arrived early but waited quietly in a nearby seminar room or café glancing through my notes and practising yoga breathing, and gone through to the exam on time. I haven't failed an exam since.

Louise, newly-qualified doctor

● Sometimes people panic in the exam – there are always one or two students who look at the first question and feel panic. Some run out of the exam hall. This is simple stage fright, it happens every time an actor steps onto stage, every time a lecturer steps into the lecture theatre, and every time a student turns over the exam paper. If this happens badly to you, badly enough for you to get up and try and run out, don't worry, it has happened many times before and the invigilators should be well prepared. Make sure an invigilator goes with you, and let them talk to you. Halfway through their friendly pep-talk to you, you are likely to interrupt them and ask if you can go back into the exam. When you look again at the questions, you will realise that some don't look so bad!

During the exam

Read the instructions for the exam

How many questions should you answer, in what time? You should have found out this information well in advance, and practised timings in the mock exams that you sat, but check that nothing has changed. Watch out for easy errors that you could make. Instructions such as 'Answer three questions from section A, four questions from section B and one question from Section C' are a recipe for disaster. Write in big letters in section A 'THREE QUES-TIONS', in Section B 'FOUR QUESTIONS' and Section C 'ONE QUES-TION' right at the start, so that in the heat of the exam you don't get thrown.

Read the question

This might seem like a patronising point, but as examiners we have seen hun-dreds of examples of students not reading the question and so losing out on demonstrating what they know. Some examples are shown in Table 10.1.

The key way of ensuring that you read the question is to carry a pen with you and draw a box around, underline or otherwise highlight each of the key words or phrases (see Chapter 2) in the question; examples are listed in Table 10.2. One word of warning, you may not be allowed to write on the question sheet; for example, in a clinical exam where other students will be looking at the same question sheet. Our advice remains the same though, but rather than actually write on the question, simply imagine that you are doing so – which words or phrases *would* you highlight?

Plan your answer

Depending on the sort of exam that you are sitting, you may have more or less time to plan your answer. If you are answering essay questions then you might have a good deal of time to plan. Short-answer questions might

Table 10.1 Examples of students not reading the questions properly

Q1 The following are classical features of left heart failure (multiple choice question)	Student reads 'right' heart failure, and gets each answer wrong
Q2 Please teach this patient how to use these inhalers and explain how each one works (OSCE question)	Student just teaches how to use the inhaler and misses out on half the marks
Q3 List four causes of clubbing, each originating from pathology in a different organ (short answer question)	Student lists only three causes, or student lists four causes originating from lung disease only
Q4 Doctors make populations less healthy – discuss (essay question)	Student only gives one point of view (so does not 'discuss'). Student focuses on health policy (and not 'doctors'). Student focuses on treatment of disease ('health' does not only refer to the absence of disease)
Q5 This patient complains of intermittent yellowing of the skin, please conduct an abdominal examination and present your findings to the examiner – you have 5 minutes (clinical examination/OSCE question)	Student spends 4 minutes trying to take a history from the patient (no marks) and only manages a very brief examination, and doesn't have time to present

Table 10.2 Examples of highlighting key points in exam questions

Q1 The following are <u>classical features</u> of <u>left</u> heart failure
Q2 Please <u>teach</u> this patient how to use these inhalers and <u>explain</u> how each one works
Q3 List <u>four</u> causes of <u>clubbing</u>, each originating from pathology in a <u>different organ</u>
Q4 <u>Doctors</u> make <u>populations</u> less <u>healthy – discuss</u>
Q5 This patient complains of intermittent yellowing of the skin, please conduct an <u>abdominal examination</u> and <u>present your findings</u> to the examiner – you have 5 minutes.

warrant a minute of planning and in clinical examinations you might have only a few moments for planning (for example, when introducing yourself and gaining consent in an Objective Structured Clinical Examination (OSCE) you might add in the plan '. . . I would like to run through how to use these inhalers and also cover how each one works . . . Is that OK with you? . . .' We will cover planning in more depth when talking about each exam format, but the key point is that you should avoid leaping into an answer without having some idea how you will go about that answer.

Manage your time carefully

One of the commonest errors in exams is running out of time and so not answering every question. You must be rigorous with your timing. For multiple choice questions, missing out 10% of the questions because you run out of time will drop your final mark by up to 10%. Not answering one of four essay questions will drop your final mark by 25%; the maths is easy, but people still do it. Two problems lead to students not finishing in time. One is planning: we would recommend that you write key time points into different parts of the question paper (we have called these '**time-posts**', and that you practise your timing in mock exams. The second reason is a strong desire to write a perfect answer. Look at the example below: most marks ('easy marks') are gained in the first half or two-thirds of the time spent on each question, after that additional marks become increasingly more costly (in terms of time) to gain.

> Imagine that you have 10 minutes to write about the clinical presentation of myocardial infarction (a heart attack), which will give you 10 points. This is one of 10 short answer questions that you have to answer.
>
> You might plan to answer the question under the headings of 'classical presentation' and 'non-classical presentation'. Within 5 minutes you write about classical presentations and gain six easy marks. Having written all the obvious things, gaining additional marks starts to take more time. Over the next 2 minutes you gain a further mark, and then over the last 3 minutes you get one more mark.
>
> In 10 minutes you have scored 8/10 and it is time to move on. You could stay on this question, wracking your brain, but it might take another 5 minutes to get up to 9/10, by which time you have lost out on the opportunity of getting the six 'easy' marks on the next question.
>
> 8/10 on all 10 questions gives 80%. 9/10 on seven questions and 0/10 on the remaining three (ran out of time) gives 63%.

You have to be tough with yourself on the timing, when you are out of time for that question move on. You can always come back to it at the end if you have time. Note that even if you don't know much about the answer to a question, you are better off making a stab at it and getting maybe half marks for that question than spending that time on a question that you know more about and getting perhaps one additional mark. *Answer all the questions that you are supposed to answer.*

After the exam

Many students loiter outside the exam hall talking about the questions. This helps some students let off steam, but for others, watching a colleague look through the books and punch the air saying 'Yes, another one I got right!'

every minute or so can be irritating at best and disastrous for self-confidence for the next exam at worst. So you might want to walk away and treat yourself to something nice.

At some point on the same day of the exam, find some time to sit down and write some reflections – what went well, what helped, what didn't go so well and what led up to this. From these reflections write down a plan for preparing for the next exams, and stick to it. It might be something simple like bringing an extra pencil, or something as insightful as Louise's example above. You might want to share your ideas with other students in your study group. They might have some additional ideas that would be useful to you, and yours might well be useful to them. The key message here is to learn from experience, and to continue to improve.

Messages from the other side

We, the authors, as examiners, have four key messages to share with you. Believe them or not (and you won't believe them all), they remain true and relevant. They relate to the purpose of the assessment, the motivations of the examiners, having some empathy for the examiners and the noble art of question spotting.

Know why you are being assessed

Assessment has various purposes. These include acting as a hurdle (to ensure that you know enough to progress into the second year, or that you are skilled, knowledgeable and safe enough to graduate as a doctor), to provide you with feedback (for example to help your academic writing skills develop or to highlight your weaker areas to you), to provide feedback on the course (if three-quarters of the year don't know the names of the valves of the heart, there is probably something wrong with the course rather than the students).

Students often lose the focus of knowing why they are being assessed. Most institutions' final exams are focused on ensuring that graduates are knowledgeable enough, skilled enough and safe enough to become first year junior doctors. Some students think that *finals* are much *much more*, and try and study up to some hyper-advanced level and as a result might have trouble covering all the bases. More worryingly, some students think that finals are *much less*, and their focus is just on finding a 'trick' to passing the exam, to 'performing' well on the day, to learning just the topics that they think will come up. These students, usually not ready to be doctors, tend to do badly. We have discussed depth versus breadth in your studying elsewhere in this book (Chapter 2), knowing the purpose of the assessment will guide you in your judgement of how to decide how deep to go in your preparation for an exam.

Examiners are out to help

Contrary to popular belief, examiners are really, honestly *not* out to get you. A huge amount of effort is put into trying to make the exam as fair as possible, trying to spot every single way that a student might get the wrong end of the stick and working out ways to prevent this from happening. If a question just asks you to list four causes of something, there really will be no marks for a fifth cause, and the examiners really don't want you to list all the treatments too. There really are no hidden messages and things to read between the lines.

The examiners truly want you to pass, to do well. They will try hard to get the best out of you in order to help you get the best possible marks. Ironically this might include asking you difficult, sometimes impossible questions to see how you go about trying to answer them. You might find these challenging questions 'unfair', but give them your best shot, you might be surprised by the results.

Transference

Transference is a term from clinical psychology whereby a patient assumes that their therapist or doctor is feeling the same as them at a given time. You will be aware of this from your own life. Whenever you have been embarrassed, you probably assumed that the rest of the world was embarrassed too. Buying condoms for the first time from a chemist or supermarket is a good example. You are likely to feel that everyone is looking at you, that the person behind the till is thinking something about you, whereas, of course, although this might be the first time you have ever bought condoms, this is the ten-thousandth time that they have sold them, and they are unlikely to even be consciously aware of the fact.

The same happens in exams: students enter the exam room very anxious and in a hypersensitive state of awareness. For these students, everything is directed at them. An examiner yawns, and this is a personal message aimed at the student (in reality the examiner was up all night with a new baby, and has just sat through 99 other students performing the same skill, over and over again, on a hot summer's day). Because of this transference, many students can be thrown in the exam, their anxiety levels spiralling out of control.

The key to control is recognition. If you know that the feeling in your gut is just transference, that everyone around you is as anxious as you are, then you can smile and let it pass. If ever you get the chance to be an examiner yourself, even for a mock exam, jump at the chance. Understanding the examiner's perspective is hugely valuable.

My medical school put on a mock OSCE where I played the candidate, and in the second half I was an examiner. I didn't expect it, but I learnt much more from being an examiner.

Tuan, fourth-year medical student

Examiners are only human too

Examining is often tediously boring. Marking essay after essay on the same topic; or trying to spot key points in short-answer question, after short-answer question; or listening to 150 students in a day ask a simulated patient how much alcohol he drinks, and whether he has ever thought of cutting down, just isn't fun. If you know this, if you can put yourself in the examiners' shoes, then you can make their life easier, and in doing so help them to spot the marks that you deserve.

Make sure that your answers are easy to follow. If your handwriting is terrible, work on improving it and write key points in capitals so that they stand out. Consider two responses to the following short-answer question.

Q6 Describe the initial clinical presentations of myocardial infarction (a heart attack), (10 points)

CLASSICAL PRESENTATION
Symptoms
- Chest pain – classically CRUSHING, CENTRAL, may RADIATE to left arm or chin. NOT RELIEVED by nitrates or rest.
- Associated symptoms – SWEATING, NAUSEA, VOMITING, collapse, breathlessness
- Past history – may have past history of ANGINA, or OTHER CARDIOVASCULAR RISK FACTORS (cholesterol, raised blood pressure, arterial disease)

Signs
- May look GENERALLY UNWELL – sweaty, tachycardia, in pain
- BLOOD PRESSURE up or down or normal
- May present with CARDIAC ARREST

ATYPICAL PRESENTATIONS
- Atypical chest pain ('indigestion')
- FEVER +/– HEART FAILURE about 12 hours post MI
- CARDIAC ARREST
- ASYMPTOMATIC MYOCARDIAL INFARCTION – found at screening at some later date

Myocardial infarction can present with chest pain, not relieved by glyceryl trinitrate. Sometimes there might be no pain. Patients might vomit, and often look generally unwell. The pain may or may not be present and may be confused with indigestion. It is classically central and radiates to the left arm or chin and may be described as crushing, although sometimes there might be no pain. History gained from the patient or their relatives might be suggestive of an increase in cardiovascular risk factors, and sometimes blood tests would have revealed a raised cholesterol in the past or raised blood pressure or angina. Blood pressure at the time of myocardial infarction might be high or low or normal. Myocardial infarctions that don't present might present late with fever or sometimes heart failure.

Imagine that you are marking both these answers, and that you have a marking scheme that lists all the key words that would earn the candidate a mark (and will probably rather look like the answer on the left). The candidate on the left, therefore, has made your life easy, and it is simple to tick each key point. It is much harder to spot the marks in the script on the right.

Question spotting and blueprinting

As a student one of the authors spent many hours looking through past papers for recurring themes and patterns, making charts and graphs and trying to second-guess the examiners. If a topic tended to come up every other year and didn't come up last year, it would surely come up this year. This is a common pastime amongst medical students, with days or weeks wasted trying to predict the future. Some graduate and go on to play the stock market, producing similar graphs of share prices, but most of us learned sooner or later that it was pointless!

When setting the content of an exam, examiners go through a process called blueprinting. In this process they look at the content of the curriculum and ensure that the exam (or exams) samples a wide range of the curriculum that is expected to have been covered by this stage of your training. The blueprint puts a little more weight on important things, so more questions will fall into this category, but the blueprint ensures that everything that should have been covered could be covered in the exam. This is why it is important for you to think about **the purpose of the exam**: this will give you a clue as to the likely content.

Here is the bad news. In addition to looking to the curriculum to build the blueprint of the exam, they also tend to look to the blueprints of the same exam in previous years; they will *know* if a certain question tends to come up every other year, and they will *know that the students know*. To avoid alternate years of students not learning the topic, they might decide to drop it in to an 'unexpected' year, or leave it out for a couple of years.

Really dedicated examiners will even turn to the blueprints of the other exams that you have sat and will be sitting to ensure that there is a really good spread of topics, with important things (diabetes, heart attacks, etc.) coming up quite a few times and rarer/less important things covered less often, but still making an outing from time to time.

If you wish, therefore, to guess the content of the exam, ensure that you know the purpose of the exam, and the level expected. From this you will be able to list the important and common topics that are likely to come up – you need to know these well – and also the less common topics that might come up – you will need to know enough about these to be 'good enough' at the level of the exam. Making predictions any more specific than this is just a waste of time that you could be spending studying.

Chapter 11 **Exam technique: specific examples**

OVERVIEW

This chapter first describes the range of assessments used in medical education, and then applies the general rules covered in Chapter 10 to specific examples. Note that although there are some very good general books available on exam technique in higher education (see References and further reading), it is hard to find any that provide useful advice on the range of assessments used specifically in medical courses. Each medical school seems to add its own flavour to its assessments, so supplement these rather generic pages with discussions with the other students in your year, those in the years above, any past papers in the library and any friendly faculty members that you come across.

Introduction

It would be rather dull to punctuate each paragraph with a disclaimer, so here is one reminder that good exam technique helps you to effectively demonstrate what you know/can do. It does not, in any way, replace the fact that you need to have learnt the content first! You must also remember from the first section of Chapter 10 that you should make every effort to find out the exact format of the exams at your school. As you will read below, everyone has their own specific variations based on common themes.

How to Succeed at Medical School: an essential guide to learning. By Dason Evans and Jo Brown. Published 2009 by Blackwell Publishing, ISBN: 978-1-4051-5139-9.

Types of exams

Multiple choice exams

By multiple choice exams, we refer to any assessment when you are asked to choose between different options in order to demonstrate that you know something. These are popular exams, not least because they are easy to mark using automatic systems, such as optical readers of mark sheets (you mark in pencil and a computer scanner reads your answers and calculates your marks, along with a whole lot of exam statistics in seconds) and even direct-entry exams where you interact with a computer (removing the need for someone to stand over a computer scanner cursing every time it gets jammed). Examples of different multiple choice formats are described.

True–false items
Each item is independently marked as either true or false.

These are generally less popular in medical education as they tend to test regurgitation of simple facts rather than understanding, and tend not to appreciate that there is often not a single answer. Some schools still use them quite a lot.

Example true–false multiple choice question

Q7 With regards to diabetes

A Insulin resistance is commoner in type 2 (late onset) than type 1 diabetes (T)
B A single fasting blood glucose of greater than 5.0 is diagnostic (F)
C Women who develop diabetes in pregnancy are more likely to develop diabetes in later life (T)

Best of five
In these questions you are asked to choose from a list of five items and choose the one which is *most true* or *most relevant* to the lead in (or 'stem') of the question. This allows for uncertainty and some degree of judgement. Q8 gives an example of how some simple true–false questions can be converted to a best-of-five format (here best of three). In Q9, both items B and C might be true, but B is less clear, more debatable than C, so the correct answer is C.

Example 'best of five' format

Q8 With regards to diabetes, which of the following statements is TRUE?

A Insulin resistance is commoner in type 1 (early-onset) diabetes than type 2
B A single fasting blood glucose of greater than 5.0 is diagnostic
C Women who develop diabetes in pregnancy are more likely to develop diabetes in later life (CORRECT)

Q9 with regards to study skills, which of the following statements is most true?

A Drawing a MindMap is only possible if you have A3 paper
B The Cornell method is best used in lectures
C It takes about 3 months to learn a new study skill effectively (CORRECT)
D Study skills tend to make little difference to performance
E Copying out chunks of text from a textbook is an active learning technique

---

Extended matching questions (EMQs)

This format of questions is becoming rather common in medical education. Each question (stem) has a general topic, followed by a range of possible answers. The student is then presented with a number of question items (often in the form of a scenario), and they need to select one (or sometimes more than one) answer for each item from the list of items.

Example of extended matching questions

A True–false multiple choice	G Objective structured clinical examination
B Best of five	H Viva voce examination
C Extended matching questions	I Portfolio-based assessment
D Short answer questions	J Computer-marked assessment
E Essay questions in an exam	K Blood test
F Non-timed essay questions	

Each of the descriptions below relates to a different form of assessment, choose the **single most appropriate answer** from the list above

Q10 A student who graduated in the 1980s sat this knowledge-based exam and had to select whether each of 600 items relating to basic and clinical sciences were true or not

Q11 A medical school decides to replace the traditional assessments in the final year with this method that requires students to collect evidence from a wide range of sources to demonstrate that they have the required attributes to graduate

This format allows examiners to ask some reasonably probing questions to try and assess **understanding** rather than just knowledge and even some **problem-solving skills.**

Written exams
Essays
Essays will be familiar to all students. At medical school you will be required to write some essays, certainly as assignments within coursework, and still in some schools as part of formal exams. Essays are tiresome to mark and can be challenging to mark fairly. As a result they seem to feature less often within medical school assessments, and when they do students can feel unprepared. We have not included a section on essays in this chapter, but have included some information on essays and academic writing in Chapter 6.

Short-answer questions
These questions ask students to write, in free text, what they know about a subject. Questions are usually structured and very focused, and answers are usually given in note form as shown in the example in the Chapter 10. Some institutions give single questions (e.g. Q12), others break a question down into sub-parts to help structure the answer (see Q13). The marking scheme is usually very apparent, and candidates usually write their answers directly on the question sheet, including any rough working.

> Q12 Describe the initial clinical presentations of myocardial infarction (a heart attack) (10 points)
>
> Q13 Describe the classical acute symptoms of a myocardial infarction (4 marks)
>
> Describe the key findings likely on examination of a patient suffering from a myocardial infarction (3 marks)
>
> List the principal initial investigations required to confirm a myocardial infarction (3 marks)

Clinical exams
If you are to graduate as a doctor, clearly it is important that you will be able to demonstrate that you can apply your knowledge and skills directly with patients. Traditionally this was tested through **long and short cases**: long cases where you saw one or two patients, took their history, examined them and tried to work out what was going on before presenting your findings to the examiners and answering questions, and short cases where the examiners would take you to see 'bits' of patients to see if you could spot what was going

on. On one session you might see three different sorts of arthritis of the hand, listen to a couple of different heart murmurs and feel a lump in someone's abdomen, all with barely time to even introduce yourself to the patients who were attached to these various clinical signs.

These exams had their strengths, but unfortunately two students might have a very different experience, with one perhaps having 'easier' patients than another. Long and short cases have largely (but not completely) been replaced with Objective Structured Clinical Examinations (OSCEs). Imagine a big hall, with 24 booths around the walls – six on each side. Each booth tests a different skill. In booth or 'station' 1, a student might be expected to take blood from a rubber arm, in station 2 a student might be expected to ask a patient about their chest pain in order to come to a diagnosis, in station 3 perhaps students examine a patient's arthritic hands and so forth. Twenty-four students stand there, one in each station, and spend a specified time in each one (lets say 5 minutes) and at the 5-minute bell each student moves on to the next station – apart from the student at station 24, who moves to station 1. After 120 minutes every student has done every station, and the exam is over. Every student has had the same experience.

Add some variations in timing (perhaps some stations last 10 minutes and some last 5 minutes), in design (perhaps it is made up of two 12-station exams held at different times, include some 'rest' stations where students can sit and worry) and in location (perhaps it is not in one big hall but instead students move in and out of pokey offices and tutorial rooms desperately looking for the way to the next station) and you have an OSCE. Fair because every student gets the same experience, safe because a wide range of skills are tested, so unsafe students don't slip through unspotted, incredibly dull for the examiners and either quite fun or absolute torture for the students depending on their perspective. Love them or hate them, OSCEs remain the gold-standard assessment of clinical competence, and look set to remain so for a while yet.

Clearly OSCEs are not very realistic, and as a response to calls for assessments that truly assess what people can and do do in the real life care of patients, various work-based assessments have been proposed. The most widely used in the UK is the **Mini Clinical Evaluation Exercise** (**Mini CEX**, pronounced mini C-E-X). There are a multitude of variations in this theme, but simply put the candidate performs some kind of task, usually with a patient, and is observed and marked by a senior using a semi-structured *pro forma*. Over the months and years they are observed by many different people while performing many different clinical tasks with many different patients, and an overall picture or judgement can be made about the learner's ability. The advantage of the Mini CEX is that it is used in a real-life setting, and that the assessor can give rapid feedback to the learner to help them develop. As you might remember from Chapter 3, this doesn't often happen in the clinical environment and so has to be a good thing. On the downside, the original Mini CEX form is probably a little too generic for detailed, focused feedback in junior learners, and there have been some issues with actually getting people to fill them out.

Oral exams

Oral exams are part of the history and tradition of medical education, and one way or another you might find yourself receiving a viva voce exam at the hands of two or three examiners. Institutions now tend to reserve these assessments for students at the borderline, or students who might be worthy of a prize, although many have scrapped them entirely. If you take an intercalated BSc, you are still likely to have a viva on your thesis.

Traditionally this form of exam has been received with terror from the candidates. The format is rather elegant: the examiners ask the student questions about a topic, with each question more difficult than the last, until they ascertain the upper limit of the candidate's knowledge on that topic, they then move to another topic and work up the ladder again. Within a relatively short time, they can build a picture of the candidate's depth of knowledge out of a range of core areas. Unfortunately, the frustrated candidate, regardless of whether they were good or bad, leaves the exam remembering only that they got the last question of every topic wrong, and so tends to feel terrible.

Variations on a theme

So far in this chapter we have tried to give an overview of the main assessment methods. Of course there are many variations, and the exams at your institution might be different. The OSCE, for example, looks a little different wherever you see it, and indeed sometimes people will take the OSCE concept and apply it to something else, such as an anatomy spotter exam, where students rotate around anatomy specimens answering questions or data interpretation exams where students rotate around radiographs, urine results, blood test results, etc. Generally people rename these exams anything that sounds like OSCE: OSPE, OSLER, OSTE—if you have a bored moment, try to make up some OSCE-like acronyms yourself and put them into PubMed. You are likely to find that someone else has come up with your acronym already! Similarly, Mini-CEX, SAQs and good old MCQs have all given birth to a multitude of variations. Our call from Chapter 10 remains – ensure you understand the assessment programme at *your* institution, what it involves, what format it is in, and what purpose it has.

Getting the best out of multiple choice exams

MCQ exams, whatever the format, tend to strike fear into students' hearts. There are some simple rules to follow, though, which will make life much easier.

Manage your time effectively – use 'TimePosts'. Start the exam by looking through the question paper, check the number of questions and how much time you have for the exam. Work out how long you have to spend on each question (including any time you want left at the end for checking) and write next to every tenth question what time it should be when you reach that question. If you have already done most of the calculation before the exam, this should take less than a minute. These TimePosts will quickly flag up to you if you are running behind.

If you are filling in an automated marking grid, use these TimePosts as a reminder to check that you are still marking the question that you think you are marking. It is easy to skip a question and then all your answers refer to the question before or after the one you think you are answering. From personal experience, it is much better to discover that you have gone wrong early than when you get to the end of the exam!

There are no traps – if you are looking at a question not sure whether it means what it says, or whether there is some secret second meaning in it, just go for what it says and move on. Having said that, **beware the double-negative question**: these are questions of dubious value that act as both a test of knowledge and a test of supreme logic at the same time. In Q14, double-negative answers *are* difficult to answer, so the statement in A is false, and the question asks us 'which answer is false' so we highlight option A. For obvious reasons, most schools will now be avoiding double-negative questions, but one or two will sometimes slip through the net. Just go back to basics – look at the question, put a box around all the relevant words ('do not' and 'fall' in B) equates to 'stays the same or increases', this statement is true, and so we don't select it).

Q14 One of the following statements is false

A Double negative questions are not difficult to answer.
B Most liver enzymes do not fall in patients with hepatitis.

Sometimes there will be **badly written items** that might help give you some clues. Look for items that are much longer or shorter than their neighbours (in Q15, D is correct), and remember 'never' is always wrong, 'always' is never right', which is, of course, only a rule of thumb (very little in medicine is definite, so in Q16, you don't need to know much about items A, B, C and E to guess that they are false, leaving only item D as the correct one.

Q15 One of the following statements is correct

The gene for cystic fibrosis is usually found

A On chromosome 1
B On the x chromosome
C On chromosome 5
D On chromosome 7 and is responsible for coding for a regulation protein controlling ion and fluid flux across cell membranes
E On chromosome 8

Q16 With respect to chest pain

A Cardiac pain never radiates to the right arm
B Cardiac pain is always described as crushing
C Oesophageal pain is always burning in nature
D Indigestion can sometimes resemble cardiac pain
E Costochondritis never presents as pleuritic chest pain

Similarly when answering **EMQs**, often there are not 11 or so good options, so the examiners might need to put in some clearly spurious ones. In Q10 and Q11 above, item K 'blood test' is clearly pointless, and indeed, some of the items clearly relate to very different sorts of questions. Clearly, questions about written exams could not possibly relate to a viva voce for example, which narrows your choices.

When answering EMQ questions, there is a process to go through (Figure 11.1). First read the stem – what is the question about? (For questions 10 and 11 you now know it is about forms of assessment.) Next read the question and see if an answer pops into your head. For question 10 you probably knew the answer was true–false MCQ. Now look through the options, if it is there, write it down (option A). For question 11, you probably didn't know the answer initially, so in this case you look through the options and see if the right answer is obvious. If you are still stuck, go through mentally or physically crossing off the answers that are clearly wrong and see what you have left (bear in mind that you will need to look at them again, so don't deface the question paper too badly).

The most common mistake that students make with any form of multiple choice exam is with their **preparation for the exam.** You will find a multitude of multiple choice questions in books in the library, and even more badly photocopied, barely legible lists of questions that someone you know has a

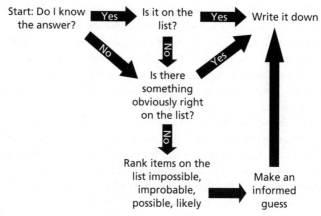

Figure 11.1 Process for answering extended matching questions.

friend who got them from someone who swore that they were real exam questions from some long-distant year. The mistake that people make is trying to memorise every question they come across. Your memory will not be able to hold all these questions, and given a whiff of adrenaline in the exam you will find that you can remember seeing the question before, or at least a question like it, but the answer, hmm, that's another question. This will lead to confusion and frustration. Even if you do have everything memorised, the chances are that the questions will not be identical to the ones you learned (examiners do not use books of exam questions to set the exams and they tend to rewrite, write new and edit existing questions in the bank of questions that your institution uses).

Past papers and external questions are really useful if you use them in the right way – namely for two functions. First use them for timed mock exams to help you get used to the format and timing of the exam. Second use them as a diagnostic tool. Look through your answers and when you get a question wrong, jot down the area that it relates to. If you get a couple of questions on similar topics wrong, that highlights a need for you to go back to your notes and revisit those topics. Remember, don't try and memorise answers to questions, go back and try and understand the topic.

Getting the best out of short answer questions

Our discussion of Q3 and Q6 in Chapter 10 highlights most of the key points about answering SAQs – read the questions carefully, box or highlight the key points and answer providing as much structure as possible to highlight the key points in your answer. You might consider 'counting out the answers': it is likely that if there are three marks for 'Describing the key findings likely on examination of a patient suffering from an myocardial infarction' (Q13 above), then the examiner is looking for three main points; unless, that is, the mark scheme gives half a mark for each main point, expecting six main points. Despite this difficulty, looking at the marks should help you structure your answer. If there is only one mark for a definition, then you might write a little less than if there were five marks for it.

We have already discussed the critical importance of strict timing and that you should answer every question that you are supposed to answer. We have also commented on planning. It is worth spending a minute or two planning out your answer: most schools would encourage you to include your rough plan in your answer, putting a single line through it to show that it is rough. If you run out of time it might still earn you one or two marks.

If you read Chapter 2 (note taking) carefully, you will have a good idea of how to prepare for this form of exam. You can build writing your own questions into your day-to-day note taking and practise answering them as a way of reviewing your study. You will, of course, want to have full timed practice exams, but you should be very well prepared. Perhaps you will use a blend of your own questions and external ones. Perhaps you could share your questions with other students and build up a study group.

It is quite easy to test factual recall and even understanding with SAQ papers. It is much harder to write an SAQ that tests the more advanced skills that we discussed in Chapter 2, such as application, analysis, synthesis. It is possible for very skilled question writers to try and test these higher skills but, more often than not, these will be kept for other formats such as debates, vivas and, of course, the essay.

Getting the best out of the OSCE

It is likely that whatever your background, you will have had a fair amount of experience of a range of tests, but the OSCE is likely to be a new and rather daunting format. For this reason, we have added a rather generous section on OSCE performance.

The aim of the OSCE is simple. Imagine a geologist drilling down to take multiple core samples of the underlying soil and rock. At some point he or she can say that enough samples have been taken to be able to build up a likely picture of what is underneath. If most/enough samples show clay, the underlying soil is likely to be clay. In the OSCE, the concept is that an individual will demonstrate, through multiple samples, that they are competent across the breadth of necessary skills, so that the exam can infer that they are probably competent across all skills. The aim of the exam, therefore, is to assess clinical competence – whether you will be any good at the job.

Students who strive to develop as good doctors, to learn the knowledge and skills required for the job, to become good at patient care, should pass the OSCE easily (with one or two caveats discussed below). Unfortunately some students see the OSCE as some kind of higher education hurdle unrelated to patients or being a doctor, and focus their learning not on becoming a good doctor, but on passing the exam. They work out elaborate schemes to 'perform well', but often will do badly.

Q17 You are a senior medical student in A&E. The registrar has asked you to take a venous blood sample to assess for anaemia. Please demonstrate how you would take blood, treating this rubber arm as if it were your patient.

Good students will have sought out many opportunities on the wards to take blood (with appropriate consent, of course, see Chapter 3), from time to time asking doctors, nurses or peers to watch them and check that they are doing it right. They will have become familiar with the different equipment available including which bottles are used for which tests, they will have learnt rapport with patients when taking their blood, and it is likely that they once forgot to write the patient's details on the sample and had to do them again with many apologies to the poor patient, and so they will never, ever do this again	The exam-focused students, knowing that the rubber arms used in the exam are not the same as real arms, will have practised mostly in the skills lab. They will have memorised a list of steps, perhaps from an OSCE book and practised reciting the steps with robotic reliability Their training and practice, being focused only on the exam, will mean that in real life they are unlikely to be very good
In the exam, even on a rubber arm, these students will perform this skill fluently and professionally. It will be very obvious that they have done it many times before	In the exam these students will be wooden in their performance, and may miss out steps that would be crucial in real life, but are less obvious in simulation (such as not remembering to write the patient's details on the bottle, or not knowing which bottle is used for which test)
This student passes the exam, but more importantly, you would be happy for them to take blood from your favourite aunt	This student probably fails the skill, or might scrape through, but most importantly, you would not let them anywhere near your favourite aunt with a needle

Looking at the two examples in Q17, it should be clear that those who strive just to pass the exam, to be OSCE competents, tend to perform worse in the exam than those who strive to become clinically (with patients) competent, and who pass the exam as a 'side-effect'.

This is a crucial point, and cannot be stressed enough. Ninety-five per cent of your learning of clinical and communication skills should be focused on becoming a great doctor, and perhaps 5% should be on exam technique. With a few tips on exam technique and a little bit of practice, you will then fly through the exam.

OSCE technique

Having said all this, there *are* times that students who do fairly well on the wards fall down in the OSCEs, and this section aims to highlight common pitfalls and give some tips in dealing with them.

Suspension of disbelief

It is likely that you have watched a film that so engaged you that you felt part of it, that you were unaware of it as 'a film', but rather that it felt 'real'. At other times you have watched a film and all you could see where shoddy actors on a screen. In your mind you may have been critiquing the script, the direction, the sound track. It was far from 'real'.

There have probably been times that you have tried to move from one of these extremes to another – you noticed that you felt unengaged in the film, and you took some steps to be drawn into it, or perhaps the film was so disturbing (perhaps a horror film that was too scary, or even an erotic moment in a film you watched with your parents) that you distanced yourself from what you were watching. Spend a minute and list down things that you have done to help you become drawn into the film, and things that you have done to distance yourself (two columns). Go on, do it now, you probably need a break from reading anyway.

The OSCE is rather similar. Students who see it as an exam, something synthetic, a game perhaps, tend to have trouble engaging with it. Students who can imagine that each scenario is real, or at least who can 'suspend their disbelief' and approach each station as real, that the actor in front of them is a real patient, tend to do much better.

Q18 You are a medical student in general practice. The GP has asked you to take a history from the next patient, Mr Leo Hill, who has been troubled recently with some chest pain. Please take a focused history in order to make a diagnosis. You have 5 minutes.

Student A enters the station, shows her name-badge to the examiner and sits down ensuring that the examiner is out of her line of sight. She introduces herself to the patient and imagines that he is, indeed, a patient in general practice. She asks him about his pain, and as he is talking wonders what might be causing it. She naturally asks a blend of open ('could you tell me a little more about the pain?') and closed ('does the pain ever move down your arm?') questions, and summarises as she goes along to make sure she understands. She is curious about his thoughts about the cause and she discovers that he is very frightened that it might be from his heart. She can understand why that must be distressing, especially as his brother died recently from a heart attack.

All in all she takes a thorough history from the patient in front of her. She gets a real feel for how his symptoms are affecting him, and thinks that she has excluded a cardiac cause, and suspects that his symptoms might be due to acid reflux into the oesophagus, or possibly a stomach ulcer.

When the bell goes and it is time to move on, the student is disoriented for a second. She had forgotten that she was in an exam. She gets her thoughts together, thanks the patient and moves on.

Student B enters the station and shows his name-badge to the examiner. He notices the examiner holds the mark scheme and he wonders what is written on it. He knows that the first mark is likely to be for introducing himself so he turns to the actor and introduces himself in the way that he has practised for the OSCE. He watches the examiner from the corner of his eye to see if he ticks anything off on the mark scheme, and sure enough, it looks like he got a mark for the introduction – things have started well. He has found out a lot about past questions in this exam, and wonders if this is the station from 2007 about cardiac pain or one from 2006 about acid reflux.

Knowing that the mark scheme will almost certainly reward using some open questions he asks 'Can you tell me about the pain' and notices the examiner moving his pencil on the mark sheet – another point. The actor says 'Yes, it is quite frightening really. It tends to hurt just here' and points up and down the middle of the chest with the flat of his hand. The student knows than an actor would have been trained to use a fist if the pain was angina or a heart attack, and feels pretty good about himself that he has identified that this is the acid reflux station from 2006, he smiles at the actor and says 'good'.

Somewhere else in the exam hall he hears one of his colleagues saying in a loud voice 'I'd just like to examine your abdomen', and makes a mental note that there will be an abdominal examination station later in the circuit. His smile turns to a grin. He knows he has prepared for abdominal examination.

He asks the actor some more questions to show the examiner that he knows the diagnosis: 'Is it worse when you lie flat?' 'Do you take milk and antacids and cimetidine to make it better?' The actor looks a little distressed but nods and the student smiles, seeing the perfect opportunity to gain a mark for empathy and says 'Yes, I know exactly how distressing this must feel for you.'

The student finishes early and sits back, trying to hear what the next station will be about. He hears the word warfarin and smiles.

The **examiner** watched the two performances with interest. Her mark scheme rewarded students for taking a patient-centred history, for exploring the symptoms, for exploring all possible causes for chest pain, and for being empathic and reassuring the patient appropriately. The first student did a very nice job, and although she seemed to be less certain of a final diagnosis, she had explored all the right areas to exclude more serious causes of chest pain. She seemed to really care about how the patient felt. She got good marks, and particularly gained marks for being fluent and professional and having a patient-centred approach. The second student did not score so well; indeed, his behaviour was rather odd. He didn't ask the usual questions to exclude possible cardiac causes and seemed to jump straight to one diagnosis, asking nowhere near enough questions to confirm it safely. He smiled in the oddest places. He gained no marks for exploring the nature of the pain, and no marks for exploring other possible causes. The examiner felt strongly that this candidate should not pass.

The actor was asked to mark each candidate for empathy. Although candidate A did not make any 'empathic statements', it was quite clear to him that she could really understand the patient's perspective, and he scored her highly. He found candidate B rather bizarre: he smiled in odd moments and although he made an empathic statement, it was clear that there was no empathy behind it at all. He gave him zero marks.

You might think that this example (Q18) is unrealistic. Unfortunately you would be wrong, OSCEs are too full of candidates 'playing the OSCE game' and losing out because if it. Look at your list from the exercise earlier. You probably identified some factors around focus and attention: you probably look away from the screen and focus on something typical of real life in order to escape the scenario, you might deliberately over-rationalise what you see ('how ridiculous, that's not what someone would say in real life') and you might think of other things outside the film to bring you back to reality (what could you have for dinner?). To draw yourself in you might try and forget where you are, by ignoring distractions, positioning yourself perhaps to minimise distractions in your line of sight; you might also try and form an emotional connection with what you are watching – try and get into the lead actor's shoes, see how things are affecting him or her. You can use exactly the same skills in the OSCE – ignore distractions, focus on the patient and try and ignore the examiner. If you can position them out of you line of sight, all the better.

You might want to practise gaining this focus. Perhaps you can role play some stations with your friends. When you get good at throwing yourself into the role required of you, perhaps you can try in environments where there are more distractions, such as the hospital canteen or even public transport. If you miss your stop on the train or bus because you were so engaged with finding out what was wrong with your 'patient', then you will know you are doing well. Consider things that might bring you out of focus, such as the examiner interrupting with a question, and practise how you can learn to manage these distractions and get back into role quickly.

Read the question

OK, this should, by now, go without saying, but read the question. If you are told to take a history from the patient, don't start examining them, and vice versa. If you are told to explain the mechanism of action, the potential benefits and the potential side-effects of three drugs, you could see this is nine discrete tasks – don't leave any out. In most OSCEs you will be given some time to read the task for each station before you enter the station, and there is usually a copy of the task inside the station in case you forget. Examiners are trained not to prompt you, although most examiners will stop you if you start examining a patient's thyroid when you are only expected to talk to the patient, and in these circumstances will usually ask you to read the question again.

Managing time

Some students are very good in clinical practice, but when it comes to the OSCE suddenly struggle because they keep running out of time. They might never have taken a 5-minute focused history in real life, or never just examined the nervous system of the legs in 5 minutes, and so they get stuck.

'Hello, my name is Peter Muthos; I'm a third-year medical student. I am just preparing for an exam and wondered if you would mind me practising by

testing the nerves of your face, this would involve me just looking at your face, testing how strong the muscles around your head and neck are and seeing how sensitive to touch your skin is. I'd quite like to do this with my friend timing me for the exam. This is only for my learning, so no problem at all if you say no.'

Although 95% of your time practising should be spent on becoming clinically competent, make sure that you spend some time practising timed scenarios. You can still do this with patients, and if you get a peer to time you and give you feedback you will learn a lot. You will feel a little rushed first off, but if you get fluent at taking a rapid, effective, focused, patient-centred history and conduct appropriate focused, diagnostic examinations, you will become a very popular junior doctor, especially in outpatient clinics, A&E and general practice.

Knowing triggers that distract you

We worked with a student who had been bullied by a teacher at secondary school. The teacher was a middle-aged woman with a disapproving look who taught gymnastics. She gave such withering, destructive feedback that our student, who wanted so much to do well in gymnastics, was usually brought to tears and eventually gave up. Years later in her first OSCE, she only had to see that a station had a middle-aged woman examining and she would freeze, heart pounding. She failed all stations where middle-aged women seemed to be judging her. She had some professional counselling, and decided to face her fears. On the wards she would tell female consultants that examiners who looked disapproving tended to put her off in the exam, and asked if they might watch her examining a patient under exam conditions (she didn't mention the middle-aged bit, in order to keep the consultants on her side). She became desensitised (although the first couple of times that she practised it was difficult) and went on to do very well indeed in subsequent exams.

This example might seem extreme, but we all have triggers that can throw us in exams. Perhaps it is being interrupted in mid-flow, or the examiner asking you to skip your usual starting steps of an examination and move straight on to the later steps, or perhaps it is the examiner yawning or looking uninterested. Whatever does it for you, learn what it is (see Chapter 7 on reflection) and actively engage in strategies to minimise its effect when you practise (remember if you are practising with patients, to include them in the deal – if your friend is going to interrupt you mid-flow with an unconnected question, you might want to let the patient know that you are practising how to manage distractions, otherwise they will think something very odd is going on).

Dealing with 'brain-freeze'

Every student's dread in an OSCE is that they will completely dry up: after years of preparation, after seeing hundreds or even thousands of patients, they walk into a station, or get halfway through a station, and their brain turns to a mush that is barely able to keep them breathing let alone hold anything that resembles a thought. Mouth open, heart pounding, panic wells up from the guts, but still no thoughts arrive.

As we discussed earlier, this is pure and simple stage fright; it is common and, in fact, normal. If you recognise what it is, accept it as normal, and learn to actively manage it, you will be fine. If you pretend it will never happen to you, when it does happen, you will be in trouble.

Talk to other people who have done OSCEs at medical school and ask them for tips on managing brain-freeze. You could even collate your findings and offer them to others. There are some common strategies that we describe here, but we are sure that you can find out many more.

- **Summarise**: it will show that you know what is going on, and usually the next thing to do becomes obvious; for example, 'If I could just summarise, you got this chest pain last night, it came on after exercise and went down your left arm, and it was crushing in nature, is that right? Can I go on and ask, did anything make it better?'
- **Invite questions**: this will buy you some time, will get you saying something sensible rather than just saying 'ummmmm' and drooling, and might open up some more avenues; for example, 'I realise that I have been asking you a lot of questions, I wonder if you have any questions or concerns for me?'
- **Ask open questions**: for example, a simulated patient (actor) has just told you that they have a certain disease, and you can't quite place that disease for the moment – your mind has gone blank. Hopefully their answer will trigger you to remember. 'Gosh, that's interesting, how does the myasthenia gravis tend to affect you?'
- **Move to 'safer' ground**. Sometimes you might feel uncomfortable or lost on one part of the history, such as the history of the main problem ('history of presenting problem'). You might decide to move on to an area that you feel more comfortable in order to gain confidence before going back. 'Could I just move on and ask you something about your family history? Are both your parents well?' This approach can lead to a disjointed consultation, but is better than staring at the patient in silence waiting for the right bit of information to pop into your head.

You will need to practise these strategies both with real patients and with friends in simulation so that in an exam, if you get brain freeze, you can quickly grab a semi-automatic rescue strategy without having to expend much thought.

Leaving each station behind

You will do badly on some of your OSCE stations. This is a simple fact, and as the final OSCE marks tend to be averaged across all the stations, you can afford to do badly in a few stations. Some students do badly in a station and then can't think of anything except that station; they keep thinking back about other things that they could have said or done, and as a result they under-perform on the next station and then the next station.

The simple truth is that students rarely know how they did on a station. Basic skills such as examining a patient's respiratory system usually have a high pass mark. Students leave these stations thinking they did well (they did most of it right), but actually didn't do as well as would be expected (they were expected to do all of it right). In contrast, students often leave really challenging stations thinking they have done badly, but actually they were not expected to do well, so the pass mark for that station might be very low. You might well fail stations that you think you did well in, and pass stations that you think you did badly in.

Some students find it quite challenging moving from thinking about one skill straight into thinking about another with very little time in between. Practise a few 5-minute skills in a row, and get used to going from one skill to a completely different skill – it can be disorienting the first couple of times.

Start a ritual that will help you leave each station behind you and allow you to focus on the next task in hand. Make it a ritual that is personal to you. Perhaps at each new station you smile and shake hands with the examiner or patient, perhaps you can see the ritual of introducing yourself as, in some way, purifying you from the last station. You might find some physical stress relief techniques to help, such as clenching your fist really tightly, feeling all the tension go into that fist, feel it getting tighter and tighter and then shaking it loose, feeling the tension dissipate (with practise you can do this subtly, and in between stations, as it is probably best not to shake your fist at the examiner, nor the next patient!). Breathing exercises, brief visualisations, there are endless possibilities: find something that works for you, and practise it until you can do it automatically when stressed.

Saying 'I don't know'

Every day, senior clinicians say 'I don't know' to patients. The thing that differentiates them from junior medical students is that they tend to say something along the line of 'I don't know, but let me find out some more information from you and then this is my plan for finding out and getting back to you'. What doctors do not do (should not do) is lie to patients, make things up in order to answer their questions. Imagine the following OSCE station:

Q19 *You are a senior medical student on a surgery attachment. Your team is referring the next patient for an upper gastrointestinal endoscopy. Please explain the procedure to the patient.*

Student C: 'Hello there, my name is . . . I understand that you have been referred for an endoscopy, and I have been asked to come and explain it to you. I must say that I am not an expert on the subject but I thought that I could find out what you understand already, and what your main questions are, then I could explain as best I can and if there are any outstanding questions I will either find out myself and come back to you, or I will ask one of my seniors to come and talk to you. Would that be all right?'

Student D (makes up incorrect facts): 'Ah well, yes, hmm, an endoscopy – well, we will pass a big telescope down your throat, erhm, but don't worry, you will be put to sleep first, hmmm, and we will keep you in overnight to make sure you are ok afterward [pause] ah yes, risk, hmm, well, no risk at all, very safe, unless, hmm, well, no, it is completely safe.'

For some reason, some (sometimes many) students think that it is OK to lie in an OSCE. True enough saying 'I don't know' and sitting silent for the next 4 minutes and 50 seconds doesn't do you any favours, but admitting uncertainty finding out the patient's perspective and prior knowledge and proposing a plan for getting the information that you don't know back to the patient really will.

Pulling it together

The last section on OSCEs has been lengthy, but only really has two messages. The first is to throw yourself into the role as if each station is a real-life scenario – read the student brief for the station and imagine that it is true. Try and avoid the temptation to second guess the examiner. The second is to consider possible challenges for you in the exam (running out of time, freezing, etc.) and ensure that as well as practising in order to be a competent doctor, you also spend a little time practising OSCE technique with your peers.

The viva

As we mentioned before, vivas are getting less common these days. Knowing the structure and format helps (the fact that they will always ask up to your level of 'not knowing', see above, means that you can remain confident even though you get things wrong).

Probably the most important skill in answering a viva is to structure your answer well.

Q20 Tell me about ruptured ectopic pregnancy.

Student P: 'Hmm, well, erhm, it's where a pregnancy forms in the fallopian tube, erhm, usually around 6 weeks of pregnancy, erhm, it can be quite dangerous . . .'

Student Q: 'Ruptured ectopic pregnancy is a gynaecological emergency, it is managed by making a rapid diagnosis through history, examination and special investigations carried out while concurrently resuscitating the patient, followed by emergency surgical treatment. The features on the history that would identify this diagnosis would be . . .'

In this example (Q20), student P has actually given more hard facts than student Q, but student Q has started with confidence (without actually saying much), has set the scene (making it clear that this is an emergency) and has laid out a plan for continuing to answer the question (he will talk about history, examination, special investigations, resuscitation and surgical treatment). Through giving this answer and signposting each time he moves on to a separate part of the answer, he will convince the examiner that he is a clear thinker who understands the information. Some examiners might even move him on after that introduction to another topic, believing that he has already demonstrated that he knows more than enough about this topic.

If vivas are likely in your curriculum, it would be a good idea to get plenty of practice, by recording yourself to practise fluency and structuring your answers, using your peers to practise answering unexpected questions and using any faculty who have experience in 'vivaring' to practise how you would handle it in real life. Developing these skills will be useful in later life for job interviews, etc.

Summary

Chapters 10 and 11 have tried to highlight some of the common pitfalls found in assessment at medical school and how to avoid them. Good exam technique in no way replaces appropriate learning, but rather goes hand-in-hand with it. Hopefully the tone of this book in general, and the section on OSCEs in particular has highlighted that the purpose of medical school is to prepare you to become an excellent doctor. Exams are part of that journey, but should not be seen as the destination.

References and further reading

Your library will have books on exam technique, especially essay writing, and some great resources on referencing and plagiarism. We have found the following books useful.

Cottrell, S. (2006). *The Exam Skills Handbook: achieving peak performance.* Basingstoke, Palgrave Macmillan.

Evans, M. (2004). *How to Pass Exams Every Time.* Oxford, How To Books.

Lewis, R.S. (1993). *How to Write Essays, London,* National Extension College.

Questions and answers

Q: However hard I try I cannot do well on multiple choice questions. I often go back and change my answers when I read through them again. Is that the right thing to do?

A: MCQ papers can be challenging. Some students tend to answer more questions right the first time, and then become indecisive and 'correct' them to become wrong answers when they look back at the end. Other students tend to improve their score by checking. Do some practice questions, and note down which answers you change. Tot up your score before and after making changes and see what the difference is for you. Do this for a few mock exams and you should see a pattern emerging.

Q: I understand that I shouldn't copy out someone else's text from their work and not attribute it to them, but it is OK to paraphrase, isn't it?

A: If you use someone's ideas, you must reference. Descartes said: 'I think, therefore I am.' Even if you paraphrase to 'I think, therefore I exist' it remains his idea, and not yours. Paraphrased plagiarism is harder to detect than 'cut and pasted' plagiarism, but is no less wrong.

Q: In a multiple choice question paper, should I leave the questions I'm not sure of blank to come back to or should I guess?

A: This depends on the sort of exam, the amount of time and your personal preference. In general it is better to answer everything as you go along, leaving none blank. This makes it easier to time accurately and helps reduce the risk of you getting out of sync between the question sheet and the mark sheet. If you are allowed to rub out answers, then mark the question sheet to highlight the ones that you have guessed, so that you can go back.

Chapter 12 **Thinking ahead: student-selected components, careers and electives**

OVERVIEW

This chapter provides an overview of some of the choices that you will need to make during your time at medical school that might affect your future career. There are some themes running through this chapter: these include consciously planning activities in order to inform your future career choices; being careful not to narrow your options too quickly, and re-evaluating your career knowledge and career position often. As always, curiosity will serve you well; you will have a lot to learn from others, even if theirs is not your preferred career. The hardest message is that you should expect some disappointments along the way; things don't always turn out the way you expected on day one. Often students' childhood dreams of being a psychiatrist, or paediatrician, or whatever, crumble to dust during clinical attachments in those specialities. Your aim, therefore, should not be to stick to one choice, but should be to make sure that things will turn out well, and that your career is guided more by active choices and less by chance.

Careers in medicine

There are whole text-books written about careers in medicine, whole departments of faculty employed to advise you. We are not intending to replace these valuable resources, indeed medical careers are currently very much in flux and are likely to remain that way for some time to come. The older systems of slowly advancing and then waiting around for the consultant or general practice partnership that you were going to keep for life are gone, and in its place is a fast-track run-through system, which will probably result in specialists changing jobs far more often than previously.

How to Succeed at Medical School: an essential guide to learning. By Dason Evans and Jo Brown. Published 2009 by Blackwell Publishing, ISBN: 978-1-4051-5139-9.

These fast-track programmes require early decisions about careers: you will be expected in your foundation years to be making some decisions about where you want to end up 5 or 7 years later. This causes much stress to many. You can minimise this stress by being strategic at medical school, and building a portfolio of experiences that will guide you to the areas that you are interested in pursuing, and the areas that really don't 'do it' for you.

The current blurb for the fast-track systems is that there will be little flexibility; they will run like efficient conveyor belts, with FY2 doctors joining at the bottom and falling off the top as specialists. In reality, of course, humans are messy – they get sick, get pregnant, they go off abroad for a year, emigrate halfway through their training, or have even been known to *change their minds* halfway through training as to their preferred career. Any system will need to adapt to this messiness, will need to become organic, even if this is not evident in the formal planning. In other words, there will *always* be second chances.

You should see it as one of your main jobs at medical school, from day one, to be curious about other people's careers: ask every clinician you meet the story of how they reached their current position, ask them what the best bit and the worst bit of their job is. You might not want to do gynaecology for a career, but you can still learn a lot from the career path and choices that a gynaecologist made. When did they know that that career was for them? Did they take any career gaps? How did they know that they were ready to be a consultant? If you discover that everyone who you respect spent time abroad, for example, then you might feel more tempted to build that into your career plan as well.

> *I don't know what kind of doctor I want to be. I'm really looking forward to the next few years and getting a real flavour of the range of options I have.*
>
> Josh, first-year medical student

Try and engage with all the medical specialties (including general practice, general medicine, general surgery, etc.) that you are connected to as a student, and if you miss out on some, think of ways of finding out about them. One way is through arranging Student-Selected Components (SSCs) as discussed in the next section, but there are other options too; talk to students who have been attached to those specialities, perhaps during some spare time you could hang around on their wards (introduce yourself to the nurses first) and see if you can shadow the junior doctors, ask to sit in on clinic or to go to the departmental meetings or training.

Some students feel awkward approaching clinicians to ask about careers. If this includes you, try the following exercise.

EXERCISE

Imagine that you are a specialist in one of the smaller specialties, let's say tropical neurology; you have spent your life pursuing this specialty, it is your vocation and your passion. Your one regret is that the medical school doesn't recognise its importance enough for it to be included on the medical student rotations. A medical student contacts you asking if he or she can meet with you to ask about tropical neurology as a career. How do you respond?

Student-Selected Components/Modules

Thanks to the GMC (1993), almost every medical school curriculum in the UK comprises core material and optional components. These optional components, called different things in different institutions, commonly SSC or SSM, usually last for 2–4 continuous weeks, sometimes lasting a half-day or a day a week for 10 or 5 weeks. They are supposed to be opportunities to investigate a topic in more depth; you might, for example, have an SSC in embryology or haematology or sexual health. These SSCs will occur throughout your years at medical school, with some having a predominantly academic slant, others being more clinically focused. Within all this diversity, there are principally two types of SSC: formal ones and self-arranged ones.

Off-the-shelf student-selected components

Most SSCs are offered as formal, school arranged, off-the-shelf affairs, where you read the description and put your name down. Usually there is some system of allocation that seems reasonably fair if you get your first choice and terribly unfair when you don't. When you look through the options, students commonly choose depending on interest, likelihood of getting their choice, ease of the course and suspected grade (SSCs where most students get As seem remarkably popular). You might want to also add into this equation some thoughts about career. If you have always wanted to be a paediatrician since as early as you can remember, then perhaps an early SSC in paediatrics will be useful to see whether it is what you really expected. If you think that an academic career in research will be for you, then how about an SSM that involves some sort of research; perhaps you will discover that you hate statistics, or academic writing is not for you. Better to find these things out early. If you can't decide between obstetrics and gynaecology or pathology as a career, an SSC in each in your first couple years will give you more information to help you decide.

Self-arranged student-selected components

Self-arranged SSCs can be particularly fruitful in helping you with career choices. The most important person here is the SSC officer/coordinator/ administrator in the student office. This is someone to build a relationship with as they will know the regulations, and the loopholes. Lets say that you are interested in paediatric surgery and yet there is no formal attachment or pre-existing SSC in that specialty; most medical schools will allow you to arrange your own, either at your home hospital or further abroad, so long as you follow certain rules. Get these in advance and piece together a proposal – you might want to send some e-mails off to paediatric surgery departments asking about the possibility of an attachment (make the e-mail enthusiastic but not too over the top), or you might want to talk to the SSC officer at your institution, he or she might know of other students who did a really good attachment with a certain surgeon:

> Great students are those who are proactive. Many of the situations students face, whether they are academic or personal can be resolved or managed, though are often left until they become unnecessarily difficult and complicated.
>
> Students need to view approaching the Student Office as not a sign of their failure to achieve as an individual, but rather as taking a responsible and professional approach to managing their education, which in turn are both key qualities which should resonate throughout their future careers.

> Mr Robert Sprott, Bart's and the London

Cheek and charm are essential when arranging your own SSCs. This includes expressing your enthusiasm, commitment and good organisation when you are trying to arrange it, during it (sounds unnecessary to say, but you should attend 110% and engage with the team, the clinicians and the patients) and after. The period after the SSM is particularly important: write a brief, honest but constructive report and put it in your portfolio (see Chapter 7). Send a copy (modified if necessary) to the person who supervised you, and consider keeping in touch with them, perhaps an e-mail every term updating them on your progress. They might be a useful contact in the future for references, summer jobs or careers advice. Importantly, also send a copy of the report to the SSM officer, thanking them for the help that they gave you in organising it (even if that help wasn't as great as it could have been). If you have arranged an SSM abroad, think about bringing back something local and inexpensive (Belgian chocolates if you were in Belgium, Swiss chocolates if in Switzerland, you get the idea) for the student office, and let them know how it went. Next time you want to build your own SSC, the student office will know that you are the sort of student who will make the most of it, and they are more likely to put themselves out to help.

When second best *is* good enough

It will happen more than once that you will be denied your first choice of SSC or even of clinical rotation. Rather than that paediatrics SSC that she was hoping for, student A finds herself 'trapped' in a General Practice SSC; ironically, student B is in the opposite situation. They tried to change, but realised that if they pushed it much further they would fall out with the student office, so they decide to make the most of it. Some students in this situation will do the minimum necessary to pass the SSC and spend most of their time elsewhere, either in body or spirit. We would advise one of two other routes.

The first thing you could try is to throw yourself into this specialty, which was not your first choice. If you want to be a good hospital-based paediatrician you will need to understand how general practice works pretty well – how else can you refer patients back for follow-up from their GP? In fact, it is hard to think of any specialty that does not require a clear understanding of other specialties. Indeed, things often fall apart when this is missing. So your first option is to throw yourself into the SSC and see what you can get out of it; you never know, you might even realise that you had some misconceptions about the subject, and it is more interesting that you thought. Much as you might hate gastroenterology, you will see countless patients with bowel problems, and need to explain endoscopy to hundreds of patients and probably a few simulated patients in exams, so an attachment in gastroenterology might be fruitful after all.

Your second option is to negotiate for a modification of the SSM. In our example above, where student A wanted a paediatrics attachment and got a GP attachment, she could ask to be involved with baby clinics, school visits, perhaps a young person's asthma clinic. Student B, who wanted an attachment in general practice but ended up with the paediatricians, could ask to do some community paediatrics clinics, outpatient clinics, perhaps do baby checks with the paediatric or obstetric senior house officer. Student A learns about paediatrics in general practice; student B learns some important skills for general practice within a paediatric attachment.

Remember, especially if people agree to bend the rules for you, to show that you are grateful for the opportunities that come your way.

Electives

Tradition has it that medical students spend some time away, usually in their final year, to study in another institution for a prolonged period (variable between medical schools, but usually in the order of a couple of months). Most students choose somewhere exotic, and combine study with travel and immersion in a different culture. Some students stay home, arranging attachments where they will be with a team long enough to take some responsibility and see practice in more depth than they ever had time to as a medical student.

Your school will provide support and guidance, and even some rules about arranging electives, and you should take full advantage of this, along with previous students' elective reports (usually to be found in the library, sometimes online or in the student office), and you will even find some books on electives abroad (see further reading).

Choosing an elective

Before choosing a country, or even a specialty, you might want to stop and think about what you want to get out of this period. Spend some time deciding on what the **goals** of the elective are. Be honest with yourself, you don't need to share this list of goals with anyone else, not before editing it. It might be that you are considering a career in nuclear medicine, and you want to spend the time shadowing a nuclear medicine consultant to be sure that you know what they really do. Perhaps you are sure that you want to be an HIV physician, and an opportunity to work in an HIV hospice in a developing country will help you recognise late complications of the disease, rarely seen now in the UK, and also won't do your job applications any harm. You may, however, have more personal goals in mind. Perhaps this will be your first time distant from home, and for some it will be a chance to explore something about themselves as well as a different country; for others it might be an opportunity to finally lay some demons from the past to rest, what better place to do this than trekking across the Himalayas.

Once you have set some goals, the possible locations become easier to choose. You will need to keep your options fairly broad so that you have multiple layers of suitable back-up plans, but be reassured that by this stage in your career you will be highly skilled at gathering information – just don't forget to talk to the others who might have been there before and look at some books as well as the Google searches!

Probably the most important thing for an elective is your supervisor. Finding the right supervisor, someone who is enthusiastic, will welcome you and provide guidance and mentoring will make a major difference to your experience, regardless of whether you are in Guatemala or Southend-on-Sea. Speak to others who have worked with the same supervisor, look for recommendations and personal contacts of faculty (ask 'but what is he/she like as a person?' to get an indication), and see what sort of relationship you can build by e-mail.

Ethical considerations

If you are travelling far afield, you might need to pay particular attention to any ethical issues of your trip. If you are travelling to a medically under-resourced population, for example, and are likely to be given a great deal of autonomy and responsibility without support and supervision, then there are clear ethical issues. You might be able to find another institution in the same country where you will have better supervision. Similarly, if you are starting or involved with a project while abroad, perhaps providing healthcare or training, think about what will happen when you leave. It might be better not to start something that cannot be sustained.

There often are not clear rights and wrongs, but it is important that you consider the implications of your elective, and that you talk this through with your peers and tutors. In years to come, this is a time to look back on with fond memories, not tinged with regret.

> I went on elective to a small hospital in Africa thinking that I would have a fantastic experience. It turned out that sometimes I was the only 'medical' person available, and I ended up having more responsibility than I could cope with. I'm not sure that it was the experience that I had hoped for.
>
> James, newly qualified doctor

Funding

You might be surprised at the range of funding opportunities for electives. If you are performing a specific project, or if there is a significant level of personal development, funders are likely to be interested in supporting you. Speak to your student office about funding possibilities, and even consider alternative sources such as industry, charities and professional bodies. This might be a good opportunity to learn how to write funding applications, and remember, 'if you don't ask you won't get' – little harm in sending an enthu-siastic letter or two out to potential funders.

Culture

Max Chevalier is an educationalist working with non-governmental organ-isations (NGOs) setting up rehabilitation training centres in post-conflict countries. As part of his unpublished master's thesis, he conducted a qualita-tive analysis of the experiences and perceptions of Dutch physiotherapists who travelled to developing countries on elective. Some students returned home enriched by the experience, valuing having been part of a different cul-ture and gaining a huge amount of respect for healthcare workers working in low resource settings, whereas other students returned with negative experiences, often with rather deep-seated prejudices that seemed to have developed while away. It was hard to find reliable predictors of a good outcome, but the following factors seemed helpful:

- having a good relationship with their supervisor or others who had worked or lived in the host country;
- having personal traits and approaches such as
  - flexibility
  - non-judgemental approach
  - empathy;
- knowing something about the country (including history and culture) before you go;
- knowing some of the local language;
- travelling in a pair: valued by many students, so that they had some safe 'space' in which to reflect on things that had happened, although some felt that this prevented them from engaging with local culture.

Aside from the supervisor, **curiosity** seems to be an important attribute for a positive outcome. Most students had a negative encounter of one sort or another – a supervisor shouting at them, for example. Those who, after enough time had passed for things to calm down, approached that supervisor and asked for help in understanding what they had done to cause offence, tended to have much better outcomes than those who withdrew. In Chapter 4 we discuss **feedback** in more depth, the same rules apply here: describe behaviours and try to avoid making premature judgements about meaning.

Michael Paige and colleagues (2006) have written a nice book, principally aimed at Americans studying abroad, which covers aspects of culture and cultural adaptation well. Your medical school library might have a copy of this or something similar. You can buy this book yourself directly from the University of Minnesota website.

Balance

Most students use the elective period to explore another country or culture, and round the world tickets are popular. Don't forget that this is also an opportunity to explore a career in much more depth than you would usually be able to, and to explore the possibility of working in a different country; both of these opportunities are unlikely to ever be repeated, so make good use of them. Review your goals often, negotiate with your supervisor, and make sure that they know where you are. If you have chosen your supervisor well, they will understand the need for you to take long weekends away from time to time.

Clearly if you see your elective as just a holiday period, not only will you be losing out on a valuable experience, but you will also run the risk of failing to reach an adequate assessment, which might lead to difficulties back home.

Follow-up

Consider keeping a diary, or how about a blog? Many blogs allow you to e-mail or even text entries, which will make access easier if you are travelling or if Internet access is slow or intermittent. This will allow you to keep a record of events and reflections, and might keep those at home reassured that things are going well.

Write up a report when you are on the way home, mentioning experiences good and bad, and add useful contacts' details. Think about what advice you would have found useful before going and write that in. You might want to include some personal reflections, or you might prefer to keep them for yourself; it's still worth writing them down (see Chapter 7 on portfolios). Send thank-you letters to everyone and anyone involved, including a copy of the report. Some will read it, others won't, but it is likely that they will appreciate your thanks.

If stressful things have happened on the elective, think about discussing these with others – either your friends or more formally with your tutors. You might want to think how you will make it easy for your colleagues to talk to you, if they have had difficult experiences on elective.

Summary

We have tried in this chapter to suggest that, right from the start of your time at medical school, you consider a career angle on everything you do, without being career driven or being single-minded in your thinking. You will have a lot to learn from all your clinical attachments that will help your future career, regardless of what specialty you will follow, but only so long as you see each of these attachments as an opportunity.

References and further reading

General Medical Council (1993). *Tomorrow's Doctors: recommendations on under graduate medical education.* London, GMC.

Paige, R.M., Cohen, A.D., Kappler, B., Chi, J.C. & Lassegard, J.P. *et al.* (2006). *Maximizing Study Abroad: a students' guide to strategies for language and culture learning and use.* Minneapolis, MO, Center for Advanced Research on Language Acquisition.

Questions and answers

Q: *I was always certain that I wanted to be a psychiatrist, but I have just completed my fourth year psychiatry attachment and I didn't enjoy it at all. I have no idea what to do now.*

A: This is a relatively common situation, students who join medical school with a certainty of a particular career path can have a real shock when they get to know that specialty in more depth, and discover that it is not for them after all. Often this rather drastically affects motivation and some students can get pretty depressed. These are normal reactions, but they need to be followed relatively rapidly by a phase of re-evaluation. Think about going to see your careers advice service, talk to friends, and spend time writing down the things you like in medicine, and the specialities that you have tried that you enjoyed.

Q: It is coming up to finals and I still haven't decided on a career – what do I do?

There are three sorts of students who find themselves in this situation. There are those who find it difficult to make a decision – they are 95% sure that they want to be a GP, but that 5% stops them from committing. Easy advice here, you just need to commit! Suck it and see. For students who can't decide between two options (vascular surgery or plastic surgery), and have had attachments in both and asked around a lot, try and find a job that would provide a common entry point to either – such as a common 'general surgery' start to specialist training or even a teaching fellow or demonstrator job in anatomy, clinical skills and so forth. For those with absolutely no idea, then consider applying for a 'holding job' – perhaps a non-training post that will give you useful experience whatever you end up deciding on.

Q: What happens if I don't get the FY job that I wanted? Will my career be ruined?

No. There is a lot of stress between final-year medical students about gaining the most prestigious FY jobs. There is no harm in trying for these posts, but in years to come you are likely to look back and value posts where you had good supervision and training, where you learnt lots and had a positive experience. Strangely most 'prestigious jobs' do not tend to fit this description. The same works for job interviews: you will impress the panel more by describing what you did and what you learnt in a busy job rather than having done a professorial job where you learnt nothing.

Index